EYE

A MEMOIR OF

CAN

A CHILD'S SILENT

WRITE

SOUL EMERGING

JONATHAN BRYAN

EYE

A MEMOIR OF

CAN

A CHILD'S SILENT

WRITE

SOUL EMERGING

L·A·G·O·M

BOOKS FOR A BETTER BALANCED LIFE

Published by Lagom
An imprint of Bonnier Publishing
3.08, The Plaza,
535 Kings Road,
Chelsea Harbour,
London, SW10 0SZ

www.bonnierpublishing.com

Hardback 9781911600787
eBook 9781911600794

A CIP catalogue of this book is available from the British Library.

Designed by Envy Design
Printed and bound in Great Britain by Clays Ltd, Elcograf S.p.A

1 3 5 7 9 10 8 6 4 2

Every reasonable effort has been made to trace copyright holders of
material reproduced in this book, but if any have been inadvertently
overlooked the publishers would be glad to hear from them.

*The author and publisher shall have no liability or responsibility to any person or entity regarding
any loss, damage or injury incurred, or alleged to have incurred, directly or indirectly, by the
information contained in this book.*

A portion of the proceeds from the sale of this book will be donated to
Jonathan Bryan's charity Teach Us Too (*www.teachustoo.org.uk*).

For my sisters, Susannah and Jemima.

My story is made whole by yours.

Song of Voice

As adept fingers point
My silent soul emerges,
Like the dawn blackbird's song
Suddenly breaking the black.

Music buried in the mind
Sings melodies divine,
Of ancient tales yet untold
Unfurled to men astound.

Whose beauty hears my voice?
What depths saddened my pathway?
Soaring eagles spread wings
I fly to my destiny.

CONTENTS

FOREWORD

Some years ago I wrote a story I called *Cool!* In it I tried to imagine how it might be to be a child locked inside a world of his own, aware of the world outside, but utterly incapable of communicating with it. He lives alone with his thoughts, his feelings, hopes and his despair, longing to escape, to break out.

Little did I know that one day I would meet such a child, who remarkably, with the help and support and love of those around him, has found a way to break out of his prison of isolation, and has become a writer, a silent soul emerging from his chrysalis of solitude.

His name is Jonathan Bryan. He has revealed to us through his writing how it is to be him, inviting us to get to know him, reaching out to discover who we are too. Laboriously, choosing letter by letter, by the look of an eye, making word by word, his ideas and stories and poems take shape, and we discover a child, a writer, of great emotional and intellectual depth. We read of his intense passion for life, his mischievous sense of fun. He tells of his hopes and fears. His words tell us so much about our universal human resilience, our capacity for understanding, our longing to communicate.

Jonathan has opened the door for us into his world, and reached out his hand to us in his writing. When we take his hand as we read, he is not locked in any more. And neither are we. We join him in his journey, he joins us in ours. Not alone any more, Jonathan.

Michael Morpurgo

INTRODUCTION

BEFORE JONATHAN WAS BORN, CHRISTOPHER AND I HAD
A FEELING THAT SOMETHING WAS WRONG. Exactly when
it first started, I can't remember, but we felt it
deep inside; and once we had whispered it to each
other, this feeling, rather than disappear, didn't
go away. Instead it became stronger and more
solid, like the kernel hidden inside a fruit, buried
and hard, but growing as the fruit grows around
it. Sitting heavy within us, it shrouded our
expectations and clouded any hopes for what lay
ahead. It felt so real, so substantial, that we planned
for it as a reality, never knowing what 'it' was.

EYE CAN WRITE

While I was pregnant, Jonathan was perfectly healthy; the midwife put our feeling down to Christopher being a vicar who constantly hears unfortunate stories, and as the weeks progressed and I passed the point at which the baby would be viable, I longed for her to be right. We even dared to start preparing for the baby; but the feeling, the certainty that something was wrong, was still there.

With three weeks to go, we were beginning to hope we could doubt our fears, and on a cold, soggy January day we were on our way to meet my parents. With Christopher at the wheel, I sat in the front passenger seat daydreaming out of the window, looking forward not just to lunch out with my parents, but further — to the time when we would be a family of three. When we would need a car seat with us to carry our child; when we would be going to meet not just my parents, but the baby's grandparents.

In front of us a car turned from the other side of the road. No time to stop. No time to brake. Only time to see in the millisecond before it

2

happened that we were about to have an accident: a full-on collision into the side of the car that had blindly turned across our path. The effect was like hitting a wall. Smash, grind, bang, yelp. All the sounds of the car accident melded into one as the seat belt tightened across my chest and legs. Lunging for the door handle to let in some fresh air, panic flooded me as I cried, 'I can't breathe, I can't breathe.'

Winded by the impact, stunned by our written-off car and scared for the baby inside me, I sat motionless as Christopher and my sister, who had been travelling with us, came to my side. Once the adrenalin wore off they were taken into a nearby garage to rest, while I chose to stay in the car, being comforted by a man from the garage, waiting for the ambulance to arrive. If I hadn't been pregnant we all would have walked from the accident with minor injuries — my sister, Christopher, the driver of the other vehicle and me. But for the unseen traveller in our car that day, things were very different.

Swinging in the ambulance towards the

hospital with Christopher, I placed my hand on my stomach, longing to feel the baby move within me, concentrating my hand on the stillness and convincing myself that staying calm was having an effect on the unborn child. After the initial shock from the impact, I experienced a strange sort of calm: maybe this was it? Everything we had been worrying about was some kind of premonition of a car accident. But was the baby still OK?

Once in the hospital a nurse placed a monitor on my stomach, and after a tense few moments she found a heartbeat. Maybe *this* was it? Wondering: would the baby now be induced, just to be on the safe side? Was this just an unfortunate way to come into the world, all a bit of a shock; a slightly different 'when I was born' story to everyone else's?

'What will happen now?' Having been the centre of some commotion, I was now attached to a monitor and left in a side room while Christopher was being checked over in A & E.

'They'll probably leave you until you are full term.' The nurse seemed pretty sure, but added, hedging her bets, 'Or they may deliver you today as a precaution.'

However, when she came back a few moments later to look at the monitor, her tone seemed to have changed. Clearly trying to keep her voice even, she pronounced, 'I'm just going to get some doctors to look at this.'

Enter two doctors: both studying the ticker-tape paper monitoring the baby's heartbeat from a belt around my stomach. Both with different medical opinions. Both now having a heated discussion about my fate, half in the room, half in the corridor. About our fate. From where I lay on the bed I strained to hear every word and work out what was going on, but all I now knew was that while the argument continued, I was being prepared for theatre. Surgical stockings, a paper to sign, and finally a scanner were brought in. The dispute was settled. Shown a black blob on the screen and with no time to process what 'placental abruption' actually meant, I was wheeled into theatre. The operation started before Christopher had even scrubbed up.

Escorted in, facing the far wall, he was edged round the bed to my head. Maybe delivery by emergency caesarean section was what the strange feeling we had shared was all about?

'Congratulations, you have a son.' The doctor turned to Christopher.

And then I glimpsed him. Blue, slimy, limp, lifeless, silent. Nurses, who minutes before had been talking to the doctors about what they had watched on TV the night before, fell silent. The whole room seemed to be holding its breath. Waiting. Waiting for some response. Waiting for the cry of life. Glimpsing that still body placed onto the metal trolley next to me like a slab of meat at the butchers, I felt disjointed from what was going on. Like I was watching a nightmare unfold from the outside.

'Come on,' the nurse muttered under her breath to the body she was pummelling. Silence. More desperate effort. Eventually he let out a little cry, and although it was what we had waited for, to me it sounded more like a cry of anguish than a cry of life. Wrapped in a blanket and waved under me to kiss, the little bundle was whisked away to intensive care.

At every juncture during that first day I thought: so, maybe this is it? A car accident, an emergency delivery, a short spell in intensive care. The whole experience felt like a composer starting a piece in a minor key, building more texture and tone, but never managing to break out into the major key. At every turn we expected the storm to have passed and the sun to be bursting through the cloud. Instead, the emerging medical picture of Jonathan was getting darker and heavier.

'This baby needs a name.' The nurse in the special care baby unit was right. It had been well over a day since Baby Boy Bryan, 6lbs 13oz, had been born by emergency C-section following my car accident; and yet giving him a name as he struggled for life hadn't been our first priority.

'Jonathan.' We were certain now. 'We'll call him Jonathan. It means God has given.' But even as I pronounced it over the tiny helpless baby isolated within the clear windows of the cot, I was considering the other half of the verse. For as Christopher and I had knelt together against the hospital bed and spent ourselves in prayer for him, the verse that had come to mind was from the Bible, in which Job, once everything has been taken from him, says: 'The Lord gives and the Lord takes away.' Our gift was not given to us indefinitely.

For days I wasn't able to touch my baby. Yearning to hold his warm body to mine, feel his breath, stroke his cheek, reconnect his flesh with mine, I was reduced to watching his tiny form through the reflection of the incubator, singing and talking to him through the ventilator holes. Above all we were praying that the tests would come back positive, indicating that his kidneys were working again, and we could go home.

Asking for help does not come easily to either Christopher or myself; we prefer to soldier on in our self-sufficient way, but one of the first gifts Jonathan gave us was learning that when we ask others for help it is not a sign of failure.

Once I was discharged from hospital and Jonathan remained in, I had so little time I was reduced to eating microwave meals day in, day out: the sort that smell gorgeous, fill you up while you're eating them, and then leave you wanting more about ten minutes later. So we sent a message round our church, asking if people could provide a meal that I could warm up in the microwave.

Shortly afterwards I was on the phone to Christopher — long early evening phone calls were our way to keep in contact while he was working — when the doorbell rang repeatedly, followed by muffled voices. At the end of that half-hour phone call alone, we had enough meals for ten days — I had become the invisible guest at many a table!

As concern grew about Jonathan's reflexes (or lack of them) and general floppiness, we were transferred by ambulance to Bristol's neonatal unit. But amid all the anguish of that first week, driving behind the ambulance with a radiant sunset ahead of us, a feeling of peace swept over me.

A few days later that peace was shaken by one term: MRI. I never doubted that Jonathan was mentally 'in there', and now, as he looked out from the portholes of his incubator, my heart ached for the child who was so knowing, so loving, looking so alone.

In hospital you know how bad the news will be by how much effort is put into the room's appearance. For the results of Jonathan's MRI brain scan we were taken to a newly painted bright room with a soft, comfortable sofa, a beautiful seascape on the wall, a real pot plant on the table and an oversized box of tissues. This was going to be bad. Really bad.

'There is global damage on both his white and grey matter. Your son is likely to have moderate to severe cerebral palsy.'

As the prognosis was delivered, we sat in stunned silence, struggling to imagine what life would be like for our son, our only child, our Jonathan. But the tissues on the table remained unused. Rather than question the physical implications of this diagnosis, we asked questions about the certainty and extent of his cognitive disabilities. Could the brain ever compensate for its loss?

Would his potential intellectual ability be able to withstand the injuries they were showing us? So, later, after we had wept together in our own room, prayed together and wept some more, a second consultant was sent to see us. Maybe these parents hadn't understood the gravity of the message; no one gets this news without instantly bursting into tears.

'Your son is unlikely to be able to walk, skip, hop, talk, feed himself – even recognise you as his parents!'

This extended list didn't burst the floodgates in front of the consultant either; rather, the little voice in my head was pedantically irritated by the idea that a child who couldn't walk might be able to skip and hop. Besides, I felt such a deep connection with Jonathan, I couldn't believe he didn't already recognise us.

Perhaps in desperation that we still hadn't understood what this MRI meant, a different consultant stopped Christopher in the small artificially lit corridor outside the ward, and uttered the words that would go on to haunt me.

'This is the worst MRI scan the radiographer has ever seen of a child of this age,' he said. 'If it weren't for the fact that he is breathing for himself, you would have the option of turning off the ventilator.'

But he wasn't on a ventilator, and we knew that should he need to go on one again, as he almost certainly would, we wanted to have dedicated and entrusted our small, knowing child to God beforehand. Calling a bishop friend we gathered close family to pray for Jonathan as we sought guidance about how far to take his medical care. Crammed into a miniscule room at the hospital, we held a small ceremony around an open cot with Jonathan tucked under blankets looking out at us with big trusting eyes. This was so far removed from the baptism that I had imagined for him. There were no songs: just the soft intonation of the service; little jubilation, but plenty of tears. Everyone did the best they could – the nurses provided a special new blanket for him to be covered in, the bishop brought a candle and a small font from the Methodist chapel, I wore a new cardigan my cousin had sent me and the bishop's wife provided a cake for afterwards. And Jonathan just kept looking out at us with his wide brown eyes. Knowing, loving, trusting.

Watching anyone suffer is horrible, but watching a small baby suffering is almost unbearable; everything in me as a mother was programmed to want to make him better. For a start, Jonathan couldn't be fed properly due to his kidneys not working at all well. So I had to watch my starving baby boy smacking his lips together and chomping on a dummy, only to shout out in frustration that it didn't deliver what he wanted; while I expressed bottle after bottle of milk to be put in the freezer. Even when he could be fed, it wasn't my milk he was allowed, which could be harmful to his recovering kidneys, but a special formula safe for renal impairment. Instead, a feeding tube was sent up his nose and down into his stomach, passing the gag reflex and inducing a retch on the way, only to be randomly snagged and pulled out by his tiny fingers a few hours later, necessitating the whole procedure to be undertaken again.

Outwardly we could measure the liquid going in and out of his body, and weigh him every day, which told us how his kidneys were (or rather weren't) processing fluid; but for all the other kidney functions, it was only really a blood test that could tell the doctors what was happening. So, we watched while once, sometimes twice a day his bloods were taken. This involved doubling his hand back into an unnatural position as doctors and nurses dripped out blood into vials to be sent away for testing. Needles used for drips would last at best a few days before needing to be replaced in a different part of his body. (In his time Jonathan has had drips in veins in his hands, arms, legs, feet and even his head.)

Weeks passed. Sometimes Jonathan would need surgery, and I found myself signing papers for operations on his tiny body; the most memorable was a tube for dialysis that is not manufactured to neonatal size going in through his stomach and coming out over his chest instead. For months Jonathan was incarcerated, unable to feel the fresh air on his face, hear birds sing, or see the first buds of spring; stuck instead in a stifling seasonless hospital. Used to the countryside, I found the concrete jungle of the centre of Bristol oppressive, and finding something to remind me of our home became part of my coping mechanism. So, most days I took a few hours out of hospital to walk trancelike in the city, passing people continuing with their lives as I struggled to make sense of the changing landscape in mine.

On one such occasion I was wandering aim-lessly, asking God, why? Not why me, so much as why Jonathan? Why let a tiny baby whose body was so ill already endure such suffering? As the anger, the injustice, the pain was simmering within me, I saw in my mind's eye a powerful image: Jesus hanging on the cross, with arms outstretched and pain etched into every part of him, the face of God behind. The words I heard were, 'I know.'

Books and sermons on how to cope with suffering have never really helped me much, but that sudden image resonated strongly: I believe that God knows what it is to suffer, to watch a loved one suffering. I have sat on many occasions at Jonathan's bedside, watching the monitors as he lies there, sometimes with drips in every limb; and I would have done anything to take away his pain, anything at all.

After this experience on a Bristol street, I continued to pray for Jonathan to be healed, but from then on I spoke to God not as someone to be persuaded, but as someone who knew – who felt it like I did, who felt it like Jonathan did.

One Sunday morning when Jonathan was a few months old, concern was growing over his oedematous body, swollen with fluid to double its normal size. For a child who had spent most of his life unable to be fed, Jonathan had developed 'well-fed' rings around his wrists and on his legs. But this wasn't the podginess of a strong healthy baby; this was fluid his kidneys hadn't been able to excrete. The dialysis tube had failed to work, and although the blood pressure machine hadn't managed to get a reading on him for a few weeks, a different method had now shown it to be dangerously high. If Jonathan ever gets cataclysmically ill, it is always a Sunday; as a vicar this is the hardest day for Christopher to drop everything and come to hospital.

That day I remember sitting in the corner of Jonathan's room with a cardiology consultant trying to explain to me that Jonathan was 'very poorly'. Too new to the vagaries of hospital life to realise that this was a euphemism for critically ill, I was then ushered into a meeting with an intensive care consultant to discuss whether going back into the intensive care unit was 'in Jonathan's best interests'. Having read through his file, the results of the MRI scan and the predictions based on it, the consultant felt the risks of putting him on a ventilator were not justified by the prognosis.

'Maybe this is the right time to call it a day,' he ventured, speaking the words softly, presumably out of compassion for our situation.

I stared back at him. 'Have you seen him?' I said croakily, reeling from the enormity of the decision it seemed I was being asked to make. (No one had yet been able to make contact with Christopher.)

I led the consultant to the cot. On cue, Jonathan

opened his big brown eyes and looked up at us both. Looking, knowing.

'I see what you mean,' the consultant muttered; to Jonathan, to me, to himself.

Being admitted to the intensive care unit that day was a joint decision eventually made by the consultants, Christopher and me, and mercifully Jonathan was to pull through... yet again.

When we finally arrived home after three months in hospitals, many people found it difficult to believe that there was anything wrong with Jonathan at all. The only clue to his illness was his nasogastric tube, coming out of his nose and stuck to the side of his cheek with multiple bits of tape. After all, no one expects a baby to hop, skip and jump. So, in a weird role reversal, I found myself trying to convince people that he was indeed disabled; for I knew that, whatever I thought about the MRI scan, the fact was that Jonathan was already missing milestones his peers had reached. He couldn't roll, seemed to have very little control of his arms and legs, and his head was constantly facing one side, pulling his body with it.

In addition to this, Jonathan cried. Lots of people say that about their babies, don't they? Almost as though there is some kudos in having the most difficult baby; a pecking order of adversity. Silently I would listen to stories of other people's babies, knowing that Jonathan would trump all the stories I heard, but feeling no triumph in having the unhappiest baby I had ever known.

There were times when the crying was so extreme and intense that I felt Jonathan must have something seriously wrong with him – the spasms would course through his tiny body, often leaving him kicking out his legs and screaming out in pain. Surely pain like this was not normal? Didn't it indicate a major problem? So, convinced that there was something the matter, I took him to his paediatric consultant, and to my relief Jonathan had a huge spasm on her examining bench. Relief that she had seen it, relief that it would get the diagnosis it needed and would stop.

'This is the result of brain damage. We could try a tranquilliser and a muscle relaxant but there is nothing we can do about his crying. Most babies with this sort of brain trauma are like this for the first two years,' she said.

Two years! In my anger and frustration, as I marched back through the hospital corridors, I yanked on the mobile cord hanging over Jonathan's pram and spread the dulcet tones of 'Twinkle, Twinkle, Little Star' through the corridors. The incongruity was jarring.

But, while Jonathan's body was struggling to cope with his brain damage, his mind was already showing signs of cognition. Christopher and I never doubted that Jonathan knew we were his parents; Jonathan even seemed to have worked out that when Christopher didn't have the strange white collar in his shirt it meant he wasn't working, and was more available for cuddles and playing. Whenever Christopher held him up close at home, Jonathan would concentrate all his energy on pulling the white piece of plastic out, and sometimes succeeded. Being a scientist by training, Christopher wasn't easily persuaded when I told him that Jonathan's mind was less damaged than his body; not until he had seen it and tested it for himself.

One day, when Jonathan was about nine months old, Christopher had him in the study on his lap, and I was called in from doing some chores.

'Look at this.' Christopher then proceeded to open Jonathan's hand and do 'round and round the garden' on his palm. Before he moved up his arm, Jonathan was tensing, already letting out a chuckle. 'He's anticipating it, before it happens. This is significant.'

It wasn't exactly part of the NHS milestone chart, but Jonathan was showing signs, like this one, that he could understand and make sense of the world around him.

But physically, Jonathan's life was a struggle. Quite apart from the emerging picture of cerebral palsy, there was also the sickness resulting from kidney failure. Not half a day would pass without Jonathan being violently sick — we started mopping this up with little muslin squares, but quickly progressed to carrying absorbent white towels with us. After an hour of holding up a syringe full of liquid that slowly made its way into his tummy via his nasal tube, it was heartbreaking to watch it all come so dramatically out again, leaving him weak and tired, crying with the misery of it all.

Sifting through memories of Jonathan's early life, I remember endless visits to hospital – for appointments, for treatment and for emergency admissions. With Jonathan's overall health being poor, his condition could change very quickly from stable to needing urgent medical attention. On top of this, for nearly two years he travelled up and down the motorway to the hospital in Bristol for kidney dialysis. These trips happened two to three times a week; I usually took him myself, but once a week he went with a nurse from a local charity.

One particular day stands out. It was doubly memorable as I was 36 weeks pregnant with our second child, Susannah.

It was one of the nurse's days. I waved her and

Jonathan off, then got on with household jobs and a much-needed rest. I hadn't been home from shopping for long before my mobile rang.

'Chantal, you need to get to the hospital — Jonathan's collapsed on dialysis.' Usually so upbeat, the nurse sounded quiet and shaken, with an urgent edge to her voice.

'But he's going to be OK?' Jonathan had been ill but had rallied so many times, I assumed I would get the answer I expected.

'I'm sorry, Chantal. Just come to the hospital.'

Standing frozen in the hallway, I attempted to recount this to Christopher, who was starting a meeting in our sitting room with someone I hadn't met before. Whenever I get bad news, I always feel like someone has pulled a plug inside me; I feel the colour draining from my face until my legs weaken and buckle. Leaving our house to be locked up by the person who had just arrived for the meeting, Christopher ran back in to collect his wallet. We left behind the chaos of unfinished work, unpacked groceries and an unstarted cafetière of coffee for the uncertainty of hospital.

As Christopher drove, the hospital rang again. 'Keep driving, but we are asking the police to intercept you and bring you to the hospital, as given the urgency Christopher may not be in the best state to drive.'

So now, with Christopher driving to Bristol, I was on the lookout for a police car while simultaneously trying to keep the hospital on the phone with a barrage of queries about Jonathan's oxygen saturations. I needed to hear his vital statistics because I had worked out that while the hospital could tell me a precise number, I would know that he was still alive. At the point where the numbers stopped coming, there would be no longer any need to hurry; Jonathan's fight would be over.

Just before we got onto the motorway I spotted a police car, and assuming this was the escort the hospital had promised, we flagged it down to a bus stop. But the policeman knew nothing about this crazy couple with the stressed-out driver and the heavily pregnant passenger insisting he drive them right away to Bristol, and was reluctant to do anything about it. I begged Christopher to continue driving, but by now his hands were shaking. We sat at the mercy of a phone call between the consultant and the policeman and waited for clearance.

Travelling at 140 miles an hour down the motorway in the back of a police car, it felt weirdly like all the other cars had stopped to let us pass. Junctions shot past the window. We were silent, holding onto our hope, praying, and even wondering whether this had happened now because we could only cope with one child.

Bursting into intensive care, we raced over to Jonathan's bed, unsure of what would meet us. Jonathan opened his big wide eyes and smiled a hello to me, but when he saw Daddy he looked like the cat that got the cream — Daddy was here as well, and it wasn't even his day off!

Although he was delighted to see us and we had managed to time our arrival with a brief relapse after the initial crisis, Jonathan was still critically ill; he needed to be ventilated and sedated while his body recovered from his very serious collapse.

While three-year-old Jonathan was in intensive care, I was becoming increasingly anxious about the baby in my tummy, who hadn't moved for days. Before ringing the midwives, I had one last trick to try and initiate some movement. Lifting Jonathan carefully out of his bed, attached to multiple tubes and wires, I sat him on my knee and the baby visibly kicked under my clothing. Thus started a strong connection and bond between Jonathan and as-yet-unborn Susannah.

A few weeks later it was my turn to be in a hospital bed to give birth to our second baby. Susannah's arrival into the world was far more straightforward and I couldn't wait to introduce Jonathan to his new sister.

With Jonathan propped up by a pillow, I carried her tiny body from the cot and showed him the latest addition to our family. 'Jonathan, this is Susannah.'

Looking down at her, a spasm of happiness shot through him. It was love at first sight.

When we brought Jonathan home from the intensive care unit, handwashing became our new obsession. Jonathan was on dialysis through his abdomen at home, and we had to be sterile to put him on and take him off the machine. With trips to Bristol reduced to routine appointments, we settled into a rhythm of being a family of four; having trips out, going to local baby and toddler groups, all the time knowing this could change at any moment.

For most of the first five years of Jonathan's life I didn't make many plans beyond the week I was in. In some ways this was quite liberating, as I often literally didn't know what tomorrow would hold, so we lived for the moment. Nonetheless, it could also be immensely frustrating when the few plans we did have kept being altered to reflect changing circumstances. Mostly we took the decision that we would try and carry on regardless. So Christopher ended up hosting a surprise party for his mother, while I updated him step by step on the phone from Jonathan's hospital bed about what I had planned. Holidays were booked at short notice, and cut short or cancelled at shorter notice.

Of all the things I have struggled not to envy in other people's lives, it has been the ability to make plans and for the most part to inhabit each day as it has been planned. Meanwhile I lurched from one event to the next in a sleepless stupor, trying simultaneously to mop up the mess left behind and live in the uncertainty of the present. Learning that each day has enough trouble of its own has been a matter of trust, all the time knowing that there was one event – a kidney transplant – that could change Jonathan's life forever, but never knowing when that might be.

As Jonathan's body continued to miss developmental milestones, it became obvious that having the facial muscle control to form words was going to be almost impossible for him. Very occasionally he managed to say a word out loud, always delivered in a deep, expressionless voice: there was the time he said 'Bye' to his grandparents; when his godmother brought her boyfriend to meet us, Jonathan said 'Gary' (and we knew then they had to get married!); the time my parents sat next to Jonathan having just walked the length of a church behind a close friend's coffin, and he turned to them and said, 'Hi.' These occurrences were so infrequent I could probably name every one.

For daily communication we used a variety of strategies. Thankfully Jonathan's smile for 'yes' and frown for 'no' were clear, and if he had strong opinions on something we could often see it on his face. Using the 'yes' and 'no' we could give him a variety of options and pause between each one, waiting for him to smile 'yes' for the one he wanted. Similarly, if we held up two objects in front of him he would turn his eyes and often his head to the option he wanted – the book he wanted to have read to him, the dinosaur toy he wanted to play with.

There wasn't a letter from experts or a day that I can remember when a non-verbal diagnosis was given to Jonathan, but like so many other things it got to the point where his friends were beginning to make more coherent noises, forming first words, experimenting with sounds. And Jonathan wasn't. Professionals trooped through our lives as the amount of equipment Jonathan needed grew. One of the people to come and see us was the teacher for pupils with hearing impairment, because Jonathan hadn't passed his neurological hearing test, and was thought by the professionals to be deaf. No one who knew Jonathan believed the diagnosis, but as a new mother I felt obliged to take her advice, and we enrolled onto a baby sign group. It was ridiculous really, because for a child with such severe cerebral palsy it was obvious that he wasn't going to be co-ordinated enough to sign. For, while Jonathan could move all his limbs, he could not do this with repeated accuracy. It would take all his concentration and determination to move an arm or a leg broadly in the direction that he wanted, often with his body spasming the limb stiff, all the muscles pulled hard with the effort. Fine motor control was impossible. Like other forms of communication Jonathan was to try out, using sign language effectively was going to need a level of control that Jonathan's body could not sustain. So, after months of classes, he graduated with a certificate, for perfecting the only sign he has ever been able to do – the wave!

If I had realised how important it would be to find a consistent way for Jonathan to communicate at that early stage, his journey might have been very different. But I didn't; so we carried on trialling different switches (buttons of varying sizes for Jonathan to press with different parts of his body), and different positions, giving him choices to look at, watching his facial expressions change for yes and no. Almost every waking moment (and due to the poor nights' sleep there were a lot of them) I was with Jonathan; holding him, playing with him, napping with him. Between us there was a bond that went past the need to communicate – I sensed his feelings and what his immediate needs were. At times I even had the sensation of feeling pain when he was ill.

Able-bodied friends have always been a huge blessing to Jonathan, playing round him, with him and occasionally on him, tripping over him as they learnt to walk. As his peers started pre-school and our regular meet-ups became less frequent, I asked the local pre-school to have Jonathan once a week. Joining in, in whatever way he could, has always been something that we have strived for in Jonathan's life. With children his own age, something came alive in him; a desire to join in, try his hardest, get involved. At pre-school, happiness exuded from him, as with help he joined in all of the activities. If only I had thought about mainstream education for longer... but it never crossed my mind.

PMLD – profound and multiple learning difficulties. Where does this label originate from? I wish I knew. Based on his lack of physical ability alone, Jonathan had this term stuck to him. The first time I heard this, it was whispered from one professional to another, with no explanation, but it was presented as a certainty. If I had realised the significance of this one label among the many that Jonathan wears, maybe I would have taken more notice at the time; challenged it, based on what I already knew and felt about him. But I didn't.

Meanwhile, all the time he was at pre-school we were waiting for the phone call that would change Jonathan's life. When it finally came, 'Oh my goodness' was all I could say all morning. Our world was changing – even to look at, as during the night there had been heavy snowfall, covering the landscape.

When we told Jonathan the news, as we took him off his dialysis machine for the last time, he beamed at us. We had been telling him that he was waiting for a new kidney for well over a year, since he was two, and that this would be life-changing. Before we did anything else we prayed quietly for the anonymous family who had donated their loved one's kidney. It felt right to acknowledge the unimaginable pain they would be going through now, and their incredible generosity in the midst of it.

Then we started getting ready. Our support network received the email that we had prepared for this moment, while I mechanically went through the checklist of what we would need for a hospital stay. Nervousness, apprehension and excitement convened in the pit of my stomach.

As we packed our bags, Jonathan seemed to be a bit confused; and as we drove to the hospital that morning, trying to get enough traction through the snow to get up the hill in the next town, he became more subdued. By the time we were meeting surgeons and he had been nil by mouth all day, he was looking worried. For while we had prepared him for the life-changing aspects of this day, we realised we had never really discussed how it would actually happen. Until then, it seems Jonathan thought that a kidney transplant was the sort of thing you opened in the post!

By now we had seen Jonathan in intensive care a number of times, but this time was so different. For a start, we had signed the piece of paper that had put him there, rather than his health deteriorating to a point where he was transferred from a ward. Mindful that our family's renewed hope was dependent on another family's loss, we continued to experience conflicting emotions.

The speed with which the new kidney started working took us by surprise; at one stage Jonathan had two bags hooked to the side of the bed, one with nearly clear-coloured liquid from his native kidney, and one with urine-coloured liquid from his new kidney. The transformation in his body was happening before our eyes, and was also presented to us on paper. For four years we had become obsessed with Jonathan's blood result numbers — what was his renal function like (creatinine)? How high was his urea level (usually excreted in urine)? Was he anaemic? Now, in his hand, Christopher had the numerical proof that Jonathan's new kidney was working: his creatinine had dropped from over 450 to a normal 50. Tears streaming down his face, he muttered, 'It's so amazing.'

After his transplant, Jonathan struggled with pain and was readmitted to intensive care, but within a week he was the happiest we had known him. The debilitating sickness had stopped literally overnight; he had enjoyed his first bath with his sister, who was now eight months old (before this,

his dialysis dressing couldn't get wet), and he had enjoyed tastes of food high in potassium that were previously forbidden. Despite this new freedom, now we were home he started to cry whenever he was laid down. I had a sixth sense that he was struggling to breathe, but hoped I was mistaken.

Once his high temperature was confirmed, there was nothing for it but to go back to the children's hospital. Being on very strong immuno-suppressant medication to prevent his body rejecting the foreign body part also meant that Jonathan was more susceptible to infections. The respiratory virus that he had contracted escalated fairly rapidly and within the week he found himself back in intensive care, by which time I had also picked up a strain of the same bug and was not allowed into the hospital until I'd been clear for 48 hours. If I hadn't had Susannah to look after, the wait would have been unbearable, knowing Jonathan was getting increasingly ill in intensive care and not being there with him. Ringing his bedside three times a day, the receiver was pressed to his ear and I spoke words of encouragement to him, but he could never reply beyond a whimper. I felt torn in two.

During the 44th of my 48 hours away from the hospital I received a phone call saying that they would make an exception for me to enter the room where Jonathan was an inpatient, so that I could say goodbye to him before he was put on a ventilator. Jonathan's lung function had deteriorated to a point where this was essential to try and save his life. No one knew, when I said that goodbye, whether it would be the last.

There have been many times when Jonathan has teetered on the edge. Once we started counting, but soon gave up as the admissions continued. This time it really could have gone either way: the procedure, putting a tube down into Jonathan's lungs, was risky and delicate. Interrupting our loving farewells, the consultant had to act quickly, and set to work.

We watched as the consultant expertly inserted the tube into Jonathan's mouth. The numbers on the monitors plummeted before our eyes, indicating that his heart rate and oxygen saturations were going through the floor. Aided by two doctors, the consultant requested instruments in a hushed, calm tone, and soon stabilised him.

'That was extraordinary. I have never ventilated a child in a room where there is so much peace,' said the consultant, as he finished work. He seemed genuinely struck by what had happened. We had felt it too – but we were not surprised. Having sat watching him we had both prayed; prayed for the consultant's steady hands, prayed for Jonathan, prayed that he would feel no pain. We all felt a peace that passed all understanding.

Next morning, I returned to the ward to discover every intensive care consultant (intensivist) crammed into Jonathan's room. Heart sinking, I knew this could only mean one thing.

'Jonathan, I can't believe you're having a party and you haven't invited me,' I joked as I entered; for at times of profound concern, humour seems to be the coping mechanism that comes the easiest.

'Your son is very ill,' one of the consultants said soberly, putting the intense back into intensivist. 'We have put him into an induced coma and increased the ventilator to the maximum of what it can achieve. It will now be a question of waiting to see whether he survives the next 24 hours.'

Getting into bed with Jonathan I hauled his inert, heavy body onto mine, and held him close; I sang to him, read to him, chatted to him. There was not a flicker of recognition, but the nurse said sometimes people can hear even when they are very heavily sedated, as Jonathan was. Most of all I cuddled his warm body. But I wasn't ready to say goodbye to him.

'You've got to give him permission to go, darling,' Christopher softly ventured, later that morning. Deep in my heart I knew he was right, knew it wasn't for me to cling on to Jonathan, knew he wasn't mine to hold on to. Yet every part of me was screaming, 'No, I'm not ready for this. He can't go now.'

Drawing myself down to Jonathan's soft ear, I whispered to him, 'Jonathan, we love you. If you want to go, you can go, but if you want to stay we would love to spend more time with you.'

It was the hardest thing I have ever done.

Later I began to understand the impact those words had on him, on his future and on me.

He survived. Jonathan: that's why we had given him the name, meaning 'God has given'. God had given him to us once again.

Since that admission there have been more, occasionally with stays back in intensive care. Usually these trips precipitate conversations about Jonathan's quality of life, for those are the times when his body is at its most ill. And his body doesn't look well at the best of times.

If Jonathan's life was defined by the illnesses he has, then I could understand the questions. But it isn't. For us as a family, quality of life is defined by living life with those elements that mean the most to us – for Jonathan this is his faith, time with his family, time with his friends. We have always tried to be guided by him, and have tried to make decisions regarding his medical care that reflect our belief: we will not keep going just for the sake of it.

On more than one occasion we have been asked to evaluate his quality of life with consultants and healthcare professionals, in a bid to draw up plans for different scenarios. None of this is easy. Navigating a path in our son's best interests, where the view ahead of us has been obscured with unknowns, has not been straightforward. We try to reflect on his quality of life at these times, and also our belief that this life is not the end. These decisions are not taken alone. Trusted medical staff, who have travelled the journey with other families, have been a great source of knowledge, but our main source of strength comes from one who knows the future better than anyone.

Looking round the special school that Jonathan started attending when he was four, we met a boy with blond hair and alert, alive eyes; instinctively I felt that Jonathan would get on with Will. I was right. Will and Jonathan were yoked with the same label, PMLD, and became the best of friends. I also had an instinctively good feeling about the teacher who showed us around, and so it proved. The variety and entertaining fun she put into lessons during that first year made Jonathan spark into life.

After his first Christmas at special school, we were delighted and deeply grateful that our village primary school welcomed Jonathan for one afternoon a week to spend time with his able-bodied peers. It seemed that Jonathan's education was sorted out – a special school, plus some social interaction in mainstream school. A great balance.

Yet, as reception turned into Year 1, and Year 1 turned into Year 2, there was a creeping sense of disappointment; for while Jonathan's friends at primary school were engaged in more academic lessons, time at the special school seemed to be standing still, an educational stalemate – groundhog day! It felt to us that there was no progression of learning from one year to the next, and the inspirational teacher we had warmed to was now on long-term sick leave, although she did come in for part of that year and spent some time with Jonathan on a one-to-one basis.

On one such occasion she met me in school

when I came to collect Jonathan to say that she had been showing him words that began with different letters of the alphabet.

'When I showed him "Mummy" and "Daddy" he was consistent at looking at "Mummy" when I asked him which one began with "M".'

The teacher's excited report fell on rather underwhelmed ears. At the time I didn't really think through the significance or consequence of these very early findings of hers, but was grateful nonetheless. But this became one piece of a message, a nudge in the right direction, which when confirmed by others was to change Jonathan's educational pathway. Others included an educational specialist who visited us as part of the car crash claim.

After the accident I hadn't wanted to pursue an insurance claim — I felt that it was a genuine accident, and I was keen to avoid the stress of going to court. But even at three months old, when Jonathan came out of hospital, it was obvious that his life was going to be very different as a result of this accident. What is more, we needed help. Help with disability equipment. Help with therapy. And above all help with caring.

But in large and complicated cases like Jonathan's, insurance claims do not get settled overnight. Both sides of the case wanted to see how Jonathan's life would pan out – how disabled he would be, and the impact these disabilities would have on him. So, throughout Jonathan's early years we met experts on both sides of the case who would come to our house to visit him, and write specialist reports in their field based on their findings. Kidney experts. Housing experts. Physiotherapy experts. Occupational therapy experts. Even teeth experts. I was sent report after grisly report to read and comment on, often with a prognosis attached at the end – how long we could expect Jonathan to live.

By the time Jonathan was seven, he had a new sibling – Jemima, our youngest – and our family felt complete. Home life was very busy with three children, plus we were now fielding an inordinate number of visits from health professionals on the instructions of the court. Most of these reports made depressing reading, detailing Jonathan's many physical disabilities and making miserable predictions about his future. But, one visit stood out as being different from the rest.

'Have you ever tried to teach Jonathan his letters and numbers?' our visitor asked, having spent some time watching Jonathan interact with us.

'No one has ever asked me that before,' I said. This was so different to the sad sighing, and the 'Can he do anything for himself?' questions that I had become used to.

Being an expert in education for children with the kind of communication issues that Jonathan faced, she had already realised that his eyes were going to be his key to accessing the curriculum.

On her second visit she brought some cards to show us – some had basic pencil line drawings on, others had words. She demonstrated to me how to show Jonathan the cards, teaching him what they said, before arranging them so that he had a choice to make. Sitting on the other side of the E-Tran (eye-transfer) frame (which

I discovered was a very fancy word for a clear Perspex board with a hole cut out of the middle), she could see where Jonathan was looking. He was pointing with his eyes at one or other of the cards. Eye-pointing. If he was pointing with his eyes, that meant he could make choices, and if he could choose then he could begin to show us he understood.

So, between encouraging reports from Jonathan's special school teacher and this specialist, the seeds of hope were sown. Hope that Jonathan had the capacity to learn, hope that although his body was very disabled, all was not lost when it came to his mental capacity.

During that summer we tried out an eye-gaze machine. Every time the specialist came with his equipment, he would leave frustrated. He could tell that Jonathan had the capacity to use his eyes to choose what to look at, because he could see his eyes moving; but each of the machines struggled to locate Jonathan's iris and use it as a cursor. Each time, he would patiently explain to me the host of reasons why the eye-gaze machine might not work for Jonathan – his astigmatism, his muscle relaxant medication, the medication he was on to reduce excess saliva (both of which reduced the dilation of the pupils) – but he became determined to find something that would work. Finally, an older model seemed to work, but it was patchy, so that Jonathan could only have a few options on screen at any one time.

Meanwhile, the specialist teacher adapted a phonics (a method of teaching children how to read) programme she was writing for eye-gaze equipment for Jonathan. Using his eyes as a cursor, Jonathan could select different groups of letters by looking at them for a few seconds. Most days of the holiday I would sit with him, curtains drawn, as he tried out the machine with a basic phonics and words scheme. During those sessions a number of things became apparent: firstly, Jonathan was a highly motivated learner. Even with the sound of his sisters playing in the garden, he was happy to sit inside for half an hour a day and 'work'. Secondly, even when the eye-gaze computer appeared to be working, it had obvious limitations. For example, Jonathan could control it with his eyes closed, which looked like an extraordinary trick, until we realised that the machine was 'seeing' the plastic tubing that led into his nose and delivered oxygen into his lungs, instead of his pupil. Taking this out wasn't an option.

Very early on we discovered that someone would have to stand behind Jonathan and hold his head still so that the sensitive machine could read him, as Jonathan moves his head around quite a lot. We would have to hover alongside the machine checking it could 'see' Jonathan properly, often needing to move it and do the whole thing all over again.

Most significantly of all, although Jonathan seemed to have control over his eyes, the machine was still struggling to find what he was looking at. It would flick from one option to another, although Jonathan's eyes often didn't move. Due to his divergent squint (an eye that turns or diverges outwards) it takes some practice to work out which eye he is looking with. The machine was literally trying to work out which of his eyes it was going to follow. So we realised that the E-Tran frame was the better option for Jonathan, because we could clearly see what he was looking at from the other side of the board, and his carers quickly became adept at working out which eye he was seeing through.

Like a jigsaw, everything was starting to fall into place. Jemima was less dependent on me and ready to attend baby and toddler groups, and I had enough carers to manage with all three children. Finally, we had found a way for Jonathan to access the national curriculum – through his eyes.

The final spur to teach him how to read and write was, ironically, delivered by the special school. Every morning between 9 and 9:30 (which I felt was when the best learning could be achieved, as Jonathan was fresh and ready for the day), he was supposed to sit in a semicircle around a teaching assistant strumming songs on a guitar while the teachers had a meeting. It was time for a change. We rearranged his schedule; instead, between 9 and 10:15am, we had Jonathan at home, teaching him basic letters and numbers. With helpful email advice from the professional who had first suggested we try this, and armed with various resources, I set about writing a plan for each day that would fully cover the literacy and numeracy national curriculum for the reception year.

At the special school, for this academic year Jonathan and his friend Will were together moved into a different class comprising children with learning difficulties, who were more physically able than they were. I hoped his learning at home would be matched by the learning at school, and he would develop.

During the first two weeks of the new regime, Jonathan seemed engaged and happy as we introduced different letters and started some basic whole word reading. Although after this his interest seemed to diminish; he appeared to be disengaging during our time together, and I was beginning to wonder whether the work I was setting was too ambitious. With these doubts forming in my mind, I rang for some support from the educationalist, and her reply surprised me.

'Make it harder, and make it more fun,' she said.

'I suppose I have been doing the same sort of thing every day for the past two weeks,' I confessed, as I reviewed the rather dry and unstimulating way I had been attempting to teach Jonathan. I was getting quite bored by it; I shouldn't really be surprised that he was, too!

So, instead of paring the learning back, I increased the speed; and, with the help of some creative carers we made the reading exercises into a series of games and mini stories. It worked.

Meanwhile, Jonathan was not making the same progress at special school. The assessment tools they used at the time required him to achieve a tick in every box before moving on to the next level. Some of the ticks were for physical achievements, such as holding a pencil. Stephen Hawking would not have got very far with their assessment criteria! So, required to prove again and again that he recognised, for instance, numbers 1–5, Jonathan got bored and switched off. Jonathan's then teacher and the teaching assistants were trying to do their best for the children in their class, but with limited resources and constrained by the assessment tool, they never saw Jonathan's best. Lack of resources and school funding play their part in Jonathan's story, but I believe the biggest barrier is a lack of expectation. Until the system hopes and expects that all children may be able to academically achieve, they won't be able to.

Back at home, never again did I have the issue of Jonathan disengaging; and as I increased the pace he more than matched it with his abilities, so that by the end of that first year we had covered all the basics from reception and had moved onto Year 1 work.

Although Jonathan's learning was progressing well, we were still working closely with his speech and language therapist to find a better way for him to communicate. One day, the therapist turned up with a book of choices with a list of contents that gave Jonathan his biggest range of words to choose from so far. For instance, he would choose the feelings menu by smiling when the word 'feelings' was read out, and then we would turn to that page for him to choose the feeling he wanted. In reality it took four or five choices to go from the menu to the right word.

He would often lose patience with the laborious menu system, and it got to the point where the file would come out and Jonathan would sigh and an almost instantaneous glazed 'I am not going to engage with this process' look would sweep across his face. It was so frustrating for us all. We all knew from Jonathan's answers via the E-Tran Perspex frame that he could make choices, but as yet we hadn't found a way for him to articulate his own voice.

Sadly, at the end of this first year of home education, despite our attempts to show the special school what Jonathan was achieving at home, Jonathan and his friend Will were moved back into a PMLD class, where the curriculum was largely sensory. This felt like a huge step backwards, as at home school the story was very different.

A month into my second year of teaching him at home, I was beginning to feel out of my depth. Home education had increased in hours to include most of the morning, and having covered the initial curriculum I now needed to plan for more challenging books, and a variety of different writing genres. On top of this I had no formal teacher training, and no expertise. Through a friend I met Sarah, a primary school teacher with two small children, who might have some time free to help me.

Entering Jonathan's bedroom, which doubled as a school room during the morning, I was aware that I didn't even know if Sarah had come across a child as severely disabled as Jonathan before. But I instantly liked her, and desperately wanted the meeting to work. Late October sun cast itself onto the floor where I sat with Jonathan on my knee, the brightness of the room reflecting my hopeful mood. Intending to demonstrate a typical morning's lesson, I had arranged for one of Jonathan's carers to hold the E-Tran frame. Extra work had gone into the preparation of the lesson that morning — here was a professional coming to see me and I was far too proud to show her just how much I needed help!

'Open your eyes, Jonathan.'

It was the fifth time I had asked Jonathan to open his eyes, and it was becoming embarrassing. Since Sarah had arrived, Jonathan had refused to lift an eyelid... at all! Every attempt to encourage him to engage with Sarah was met with at most a flicker, or a sly grin. What would she think of us?

Eventually, I ran through a typical home education session as if Jonathan's eyes had been open and he was demonstrating it, explaining the systems I had devised for him to read, write, spell and do maths. I showed her the Perspex E-Tran frame board and past lesson plans, demonstrating the multiple resources we had made, while all the time the voice in my head was shouting, 'She must think you are the ultimate in a deluded mother!'

Since that day Jonathan has never again refused to open his eyes for a whole morning; he later told me it was his version of a test — to see if Sarah would believe me. Why on earth he thought this approach would be helpful, I have no idea, but it seemed that having a teacher who would get on with his mother was more important to him than showing her what he could do. Thankfully she did believe me, and to my utter amazement and relief, Sarah agreed to help with Jonathan's home education. They got on well together, and what happened next amazed us all.

Chantal Bryan

CHAPTER ONE

Song of Silence

Numbness making sensory dead!
Inhibiting freedom, fearing change,
Sanity seeping sadly down,
Shutters closing, everyday night.

Ceasing hope, holding shame aloft,
Kept like wounded trapped birds caged inside,
Why should silence drown their spirit?
Who can free their souls' aching sorrow?

CAN YOU IMAGINE NOT BEING ABLE TO SPEAK OR COMMUNICATE? The silence, the loneliness, the pain. Inside you disappear to magical places, but most of the time remain imprisoned within the isolation. Waiting, longing, hoping. Until someone realises your potential and discovers your key, so your unlocking can begin. Now you are free, flying like a wild bird in the open sky. A voice for the voiceless.

This is me, and this is my story.

Listening, looking and waiting to be heard, I spent the first part of my childhood unable to tell my story. In silence I lived behind the labels. Labels attached to my dysfunctional body. Severe cerebral palsy. Profound and multiple learning difficulties. Non-verbal. Chronic lung disease. Curved spine. Transplanted kidney. Hearing loss. Squint. Short stature. Deranged liver. Even my teeth have a disability.

For all of my eight years these labels had defined me. Expectations founded on my outward appearance. But more than the rest, the silence. Shrouding my personality, silence suffocated my identity — my very being sealed shut; with my loves, passions, dislikes and sharp mind deadened in the soundless void.

I couldn't even tell you my name.

Voiceless, I had no way to communicate, relying instead on those around me to tell you, 'His name is Jonathan.' At home my younger sisters, Susannah and Jemima, more than made up for my quietness! Like a moon rotating the earth, they are my world and I delight in them more than anyone else. Together we danced to life's rhythm, unfettered by the silence; instinctively knowing and being without the need for verbal communication.

At home, life is far from serene. Constantly humming in the background and hissing three litres a minute up my nostrils, my oxygen machine drones its *basso continuo* through my busy household. Doorbells chiming, carers coming, carers going, chatting, laughing, sisters playing. But I am silent. Due to my complex health needs,

I am never alone; either Mummy, Daddy or a carer is with me all day and awake all night. Ours is the house that never sleeps.

At one end my specially adapted bedroom opens to our playroom, the focal point for us children; at the opposite end Daddy contemplates in the relative peace of his study. Working from home, Daddy is around in our lives more than most, eating meals with us, cooking supper and popping in to see us as a welcome distraction from his busy schedule. In the kitchen our lives are shared, and despite neither eating (I am tube fed) nor talking, sitting at the table being included and loved is one of my favourite parts of the day.

Special school was only a short drive away, but so distant from the rest of my world that it might as well have been a foreign country. It even had a foreign language. Imagine the voice used to talk to a baby: high-pitched, excitable, slightly louder than usual. Mix that with how you talk to a foreigner with little understanding of the language: slow, loud and clear with short sentences and no complicated words. You are now close to speaking 'Special'.

In the classroom we sat, nine wheelchair islands, an unconnected archipelago isolated from each other by a sea of activity. We were arranged in a circle with just the right distance between us, so that we couldn't touch one another (any successful attempts at this precipitated a complete readjustment to ensure it didn't happen again. I have no idea why). The teaching assistants and teacher busied themselves around us like boats, their chat filling the air with noise.

'Have you seen Harriet's feed?'

'Has Tom been changed yet?'

'Did Lucy's home school book come in?'

'Can you believe what happened on *Eastenders* last night?'

Waiting. If academic awards were given for waiting, I would be introducing you to nine children with doctorates. Some waiting was boring, some I reserved for sleeping, but some was torturous: TV was torture. At eight years old I was the youngest in the class, which was predominantly made up of teenagers. The TV programmes we were parked in front of? Nursery rhymes with basic animation and presenters that my two-year-old sister Jemima would have been happy to watch. Presenters that my parents would rather walk out of the room than spend time watching with her. But the children in my class at special school couldn't walk out.

One day I was positioned next to my best friend Will; as he was wheeled alongside me, he squealed in pure delight. His stiff limbs rose towards me like a swan spreading its wings preparing for flight. Looking into his piercing blue eyes we connected at a level beyond words. Together we travelled the landscapes of our imaginations; outwardly vacant, inwardly amusing ourselves, until our journey was abruptly interrupted.

'Hello, Jonathan,' sang a voice dripping with enthusiasm. 'How are you today? Hello, Jonathan, are you here today?'

Indignation spilt over the land where Will and I escaped to, the music of our souls interrupted by the clanging song.

'Jonathan! Jonathan, are you here?' The teacher's sing-song soft high voice, pitched at a baby's understanding, grated on my inner eight-year-old being. Scowling with frustration, I flicked my eyes open in annoyance to be greeted by grinning smiles.

'Oh Jonathan, you *are* here!' As the teacher made her way to her next victim, Will and I exchanged a knowing glance and returned to our secret sanctum.

In the classroom our wasted school hours, days, weeks and years hung heavy, suffocating expectation with mindless activity. While I sat through 'reading' (which meant being subjected to *Farmer Duck*, the same pre-school story book we had last week), 'art' (having my hand painted and stamped onto a piece of paper) and 'golden time' (lying in a semi-darkened room watching lights on the ceiling while listening to yet more nursery rhymes), I dreamt of my invaluable education hour at home the next morning.

CHAPTER TWO

Hope in Illness
Part I

Debilitating exhaustion overwhelms my aching limbs
Tight chest heavy, baking pressure of my skin
Waves crashing, echoing in my ears
Colour draining, rising fear
Stale smells — swirling
Dragging, drifting
Drowning
Lost

'Open up Jon-Jon.' Mummy's voice floated into my daydream, mingling with imagined realms of far-off kingdoms where I sat supreme over all I surveyed. Today I was in a field of long grass. He was next to me. Silently we were soaking up the sun; listening to the gentle hum of insects, watching buzzards spiral over our heads and...

'Open your eyes, Jon-Jon.' This time it was Sarah imploring me, willing me, urging me on. Education is important; it's also hard work. Extra hard work, especially when your body is weak. Maybe I should also not lie awake at 4:30am keeping the night carer on her toes!

Today felt different. Tiredness was overwhelming. Slipping once again into my daydream, I tried to recreate the scene. But it had changed. The pleasant warmth of the sun was replaced by a baking oppression – heat that was too hot to bear. Grass was irritating, scratching, burning. Humming became pounding; the insects biting, flying at my face. The buzzards circled closer, menacing; their plaintive mew echoing above me. His presence was still with me, though.

Once my temperature was taken, the appealing to keep my eyes open ceased. Like a blanket, apprehension dampened the jocular mood; joking, laughing voices were superseded by concerned, hushed half-whispers. The learning materials trolley squeaked back into its corner, passing on its way the medical equipment table that was taking its place. My bedroom was morphing once again — bedroom to classroom to hospital room in two hours. At least I could take the view with me.

The battle was on again! Me versus my body. My mother, in her new role as general-in-command, held the ground with the infantry ventilator, securing the mask onto my face. My vision blurred into the battleground within. With the oxygen saturation monitor in place, and effective radio links established, the general rang through to field marshal consultant Dr Dudley. Following a reconnaissance visit from the local GP, the blood test indicated powerful antibiotic artillery. With the battle lines drawn, we stood our ground and waited. Of the surprise attacks the enemy could throw, the deadliest were the seizures.

As my body lingered in the hinterland of illness, I lay in my mother's strong, comforting arms. Sharing a serene sort of stillness, we were together; loving, holding these moments, not knowing if they were our last. Love like ours needs no language, so we sat with the prayers surrounding us and waited.

Just at the point where our tranquillity was in danger of becoming morose, Daddy arrived with my sisters, who burst into the room fresh from school.

'Can I eat my sweets?'

'I was on the rainbow today.'

'Mummy, you forgot my PE kit.'

'Is Jon-Jon ill?'

'But Mummy, you still haven't said if I can eat my sweets.'

Our peace shattered, the realms of reality crashed us back to normality. Tumbling over each other, their questions and bodies filled the room as I lay in the middle and let their presence fill me with love. Daddy knelt beside Mummy and placed a protective arm around us both. Jemima's warm soul draped around me, her soft, supple cheek resting on my clammy chest, her arm stretching over my tired body so that her hand could touch my hair sticking through my ventilator cap. Scared sadness and love flowed between us, while Susannah stood over our entangled mess with concern etched on her pretty young face. Pulling Susannah's stiff body close, Mummy wrapped us all together and uttered soothing, placating words that we all wished were true.

'He's OK.' Mummy's voice croaked as it adjusted out of a whisper, making the statement sound as lame as it was.

'If he's OK, why is he in BiPAP?' Susannah needed answers to her volley of questions, but there weren't any to reassure her.

'What's wrong with him?'

'We don't know.'

Staring at the ventilator mask strapped tight to my face, Susannah asked, 'How long will he need to be in BiPAP?'

'We don't know.'

'Will he get better?'

'We don't know.'

Unanswerable questions hung heavy, cut by Jemima's prayer: 'Please make our Jon-Jon better, Amen.'

Games of escape were calling, pirates in the garden capturing princesses from the house; my sisters ran off outside giving chase to Susannah's imagination.

Alone again, the contrast between their cavorting laughter from the garden and my languid sad silence was almost too much for me to bear; and like them I disappeared to my inner world. Long scratchy grass was growing over my body; hot, dry whip-thongs of wild grass creeping up my thighs and onto my torso. As I looked up, the sun split in two: one half enlarging above me to fill the sky with blinding light and heat, the other half falling beneath me, burning my back and neck. Still the grass was edging up to my hips.

Jesus' strong, reassuring presence was in me.

Swarming, biting insects were scouring my body

for exposed flesh. Finding a spot on my arm, one mosquito burrowed in, crawling under my skin, flapping and biting its way up my arm. Frenzied buzzing ensued – the way in had been found. Mosquitoes, moths and millipedes followed the trailblazer. Once past the opening they spread out, down to my fingernails, over my shoulder, up my neck and into my chest. Suddenly the grass pulled tight, terror coursing through my pulsating body. Fear gripped. Chest squeezed of breath. Body jerking. Vibrating. Fitting.

'Mew, mew,' the buzzards' far-off cry called from beyond the sun.

'Meew, meew.' The buzzards were calling me from my nightmare.

'Neeow, neeow.' They were getting louder, getting clearer.

Back in the room. Looking around me, I let out a cry of anguish and relief. My sisters were here again.

'Is he dying?' Susannah whispered over me.

Bright jackets poured through the door, bringing with them upbeat banter and a stretcher bed. While my medical history was condensed into as few sentences as possible, orders were given about what to pack and where to find it. The stretcher was a useful luggage trolley, doing several trips before collecting me on Mummy's lap – the rightful cargo.

As we wheeled past her, Susannah stood lost, bewildered by the last two hours, angry that once again I was taking her mummy away and scared for what might happen. Her expressionless face belied it all, as she let Daddy hug her. Sobbing, Jemima had to be prised from me like a limpet from a rock. Sounds of her distress ushered me into the ambulance, my heart filled with prayer for my sisters above all else. Medical emergencies have become part of who I am, but I will never get used to seeing my sisters suffer. As the doors slammed shut, my last view of my daddy and sisters huddled together was imprinted into my mind, like a photograph, to take away with me. The ambulance engine starting sounded more like the ripping up of a family torn apart by illness.

There is nothing romantic about an ambulance

ride. Perched on top of Mummy, I balanced precariously, held in by only a small strap and Mummy's strong arms, which were gripping me more out of necessity than for comfort. Jolting down the motorway I felt grateful my fits weren't triggered by movement, as we rattled our way to the hospital.

Lurching around in Mummy's arms as the ambulance went from one roundabout to another was made up for by the sirens announcing my arrival, and the glimpses of the traffic chaos I was unintentionally causing. Like a boat carving its way on a river, the ambulance left a trail of weirdly angled vehicles in its wake.

In comes field marshal Dr Dudley, and the enemy launched its largest surprise attack yet.

Memories of my time in the resuscitation room are disjointed: bright lights, voices, needles, monitors beeping. Once on the renal ward, familiarity helped my body breathe a sigh of relief.

Literally years of my life have been whiled away incarcerated within the confines of the renal ward's white airless walls; but for all its prison-like qualities, this for me is a sort of hospital homecoming, with friendly nurses' faces, the fish still exploring their tank in the corner and consultants who have known me since I was a baby. For once you've joined the renal family, you never leave it.

Describing what it feels like to be as sick as I have been is almost impossible. Kidney failure sucks most of the joy out of life and the life out of joy, leaving a shell of existence. Like shafts of sunlight cast on the forest floor there were brief glimmers of enjoyment, but these were few and fleeting. Transplantation was that moment when the trees ended and the warmth of the sun finally penetrated my soul. That was when I was three, and my life was mostly transformed. Except now everything was hanging in the balance once again.

After being introduced to the palliative care consultant, it was made clear to Mummy and me that this admission had only one expected outcome.

CHAPTER THREE

Hope in Illness
Part 2

Found

Comforted

Cradled, covered

Life's light illuminated

Stable rock, steadfast ground

Voice of peace, nourished by sound

Strong arms enfold, solid hope renewed

Anticipation of Home revived by love imbued

OVER TIME IT BECAME CLEAR THAT THE VISIT FROM THE PALLIATIVE CARE CONSULTANT WAS MORE ABOUT THE FUTURE THAN NOW. While Mummy insisted I was better and became a stuck record, asking every doctor who entered the room about going home, I knew this word 'better' was a relative word for me – it only meant I hadn't died this time!

When we eventually left the ward I still had to be pushed in my wheelchair. I still had cerebral palsy. Despite my kidney transplant, I still had kidney failure. I still needed a force 9 gale of oxygen blowing up my nose. But nothing compared to the sense of freedom at being finally released from the confines of our hospital room.

Sometimes, when my body is relaxed and I really want to say something, a fully formed word comes out of me in a low monotone voice, surprising me and anyone with me. Rather than make a big fuss, which would instantly make my excited muscles contract and stop me saying any more, and to honour the speech for the communication it is, conversations are resumed. When I am very tired my mouth seems at its most relaxed, though forming words out of the sleepy babble can prove tricky. Audible speech is a rarity for me, and the times I have managed it have gone down in family lore. As we passed the ward doors my elation made me shout, 'Go!' Like the moment you stand on the edge of an open field on a windy day, Mummy shared the euphoria and broke into an irresistible run, pushing me in my wheelchair. Then, tired from the exertion after days of languishing in a hospital bed with me, she collapsed in laughter at the lift in between panting for breath. We were free!

At home, our return was met with a mixture of emotions. Running to meet me, Jemima lunged at my wheelchair, draping her small arms around me and plastering my chest with kisses.

'I missed you Jon-Jon, I love you Jon-Jon.' Her sweet voice filled me with joy.

Lying on the sofa, playing a game on the iPad, Susannah didn't look up as we entered the room, apparently too engrossed to greet me. But underneath her indifferent stance, I know she loves having me at home as much as everyone else. For a start, I could see she was now losing the game and didn't appear to have noticed; and although she still felt cross with me for being ill in the first place, and for stealing her mummy for a few days, her relief was palpable when she finally sidled up to give me a hug. And that brief hug was as precious to me as Jemima's embrace.

Getting 'better' is the most tedious, slow and frustrating business. Once home, my hope was to see all my friends. Will would be wondering when I would be back, and my local friends would expect to see me out and about. I just wanted to continue life as if the last week hadn't happened and I suspect Mummy felt the same, as she took me off my BiPAP mask for a whole day when we got back. Initially, this plan looked as if it was working. For the first time in over a week Mummy left me to go and watch Jemima in her nativity play. My little Jemima, star of the show, with no proud big brother to watch her. Missing out. I hate missing out.

When my sisters came back I mustered all my energy to play a game of Hungry Hippos with them, and then cuddled next to them as they watched TV. They still hadn't realised I couldn't see the screen when spasms made my head go back, but their company is all I craved.

However, my body is expert at rallying itself for a day — rising to the occasion, fulfilling its promises, performing to the crowd. But sustaining the momentum is hard work, and the next day we paid the price for our impatience.

Being in a BiPAP mask is like the loneliness of longing to be outside when you're sitting at the empty classroom window watching your friends play; or the distance you might feel when at a museum watching people work behind a screen, completely engrossed in an activity that doesn't include you. If it weren't for the fact that BiPAP helps me breathe, I would hate it. Today I needed it. As it forced air in and out of my lungs I felt my body sigh with relief.

For now, I had a goal in mind. Whether my body liked it or not, I would get better to enjoy

Christmas; and determination is a strong family trait, of which I inherited a double portion. There are a number of reasons Christmas is my favourite time of year. The first is a pragmatic one; my body doesn't mind being cold but causes me a lot of stress when it gets too hot, so the winter climate is perfect. Secondly, it means Daddy-time – not the usual quarter of an hour snatched between bath time and his evening meetings, but real Daddy-time: long afternoons, fact-filled forays into books, the iPad and outings.

Then there is the real reason I love Christmas. Being part of my family nourishes me, but I am privileged to belong to more than just one family – I am also part of a family that is worldwide. Transcending age, gender, ability... disability: we encourage each other on the journey and my soul dances to the music of our fellowship and faith. Sometimes, heaven and earth seem so close, they almost touch each other, and, I believe, in the baby who was born that first Christmas they become one. This for me is the 'magic' of Christmas, and it's not only for us children to enjoy. It affects people's behaviour, making them jollier, more generous and gentler. Laughter: this is the main characteristic of Christmas Day. Laughter as my sisters literally jump up and down on the spot because Father Christmas has been. Laughter in church, sharing the peace. Laughter when a joyfully exhausted Daddy pops the champagne and family time begins.

When the clock struck midday that Christmas, it heralded not only the start of our usual family post-Christmas break, but also the beginning of a new family adventure. For the next three months Daddy was going to be off work on a sabbatical, but something more significant than extended 'Daddy-time' was about to happen to me. Daddy's sabbatical was planned; my surprise was not.

CHAPTER FOUR

Song of Voice

As adept fingers point
My silent soul emerges,
Like the dawn blackbird's song
Suddenly breaking the black.

Music buried in the mind
Sings melodies divine,
Of ancient tales yet untold
Unfurled to men astound.

Whose beauty hears my voice?
What depths saddened my pathway?
Soaring eagles spread wings
I fly to my destiny.

JANUARY BLUES ARE NEVER AN ISSUE IN OUR HOUSE-
HOLD AS WE PLUNGE FROM CHRISTMAS TO TWO
BIRTHDAYS — JEMIMA'S, FOLLOWED BY MINE. Soon
to be nine, my life settled into a new pattern of
'normal'. For the first time in our family, we were
discovering what many families would consider
ordinary, as Daddy exchanged his Monday day off
for a weekend. When you are used to snatching
time with Daddy after a busy school day, a weekend is like eating a slice of sticky chocolate cake
instead of a breadstick; and we were savouring
every moment.

At home school every morning with Sarah and
Mummy, I was planning a story about going on
an adventure with my oldest friend Alexander.
As babies Alexander and I met once a week, and
then as toddlers at pre-school, and although I
moved house when I was four, we kept in contact
and still meet up in the holidays. When we meet
it is as if we have never been apart; we just pick
up where we left off. Now he was joining me in
my imaginative story and amid the excitement
there were eggs and enemies, as well as a useless

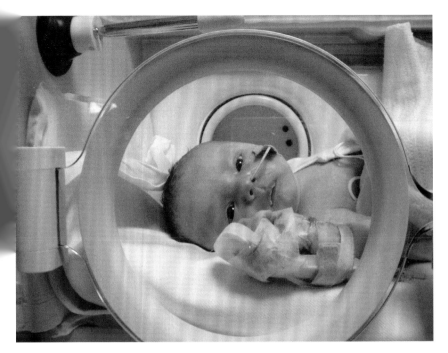

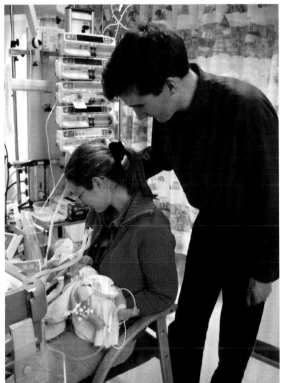

Above: Two weeks old and on my way to the MRI scan.

Left: In intensive care at three months old. Cuddles are the best medicine.

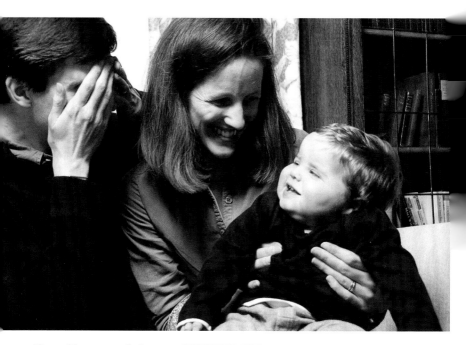

Above: Playing peekaboo with Daddy.

Right: Excited about my first day at pre-school.

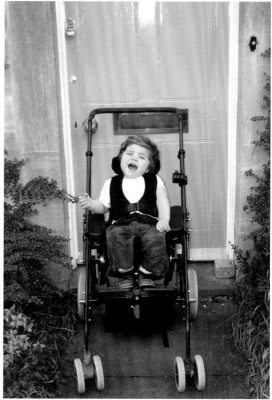

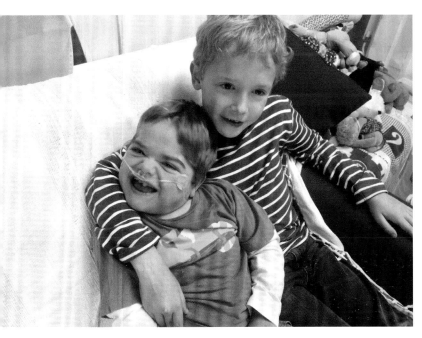

Above: With my oldest friend, Alexander.

Below: Will and I at the park.

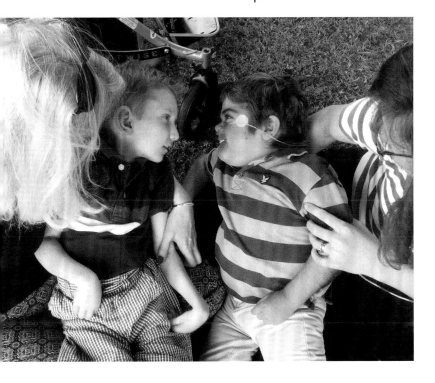

Right: My Jemima's first day at school – all of us at the same primary school.

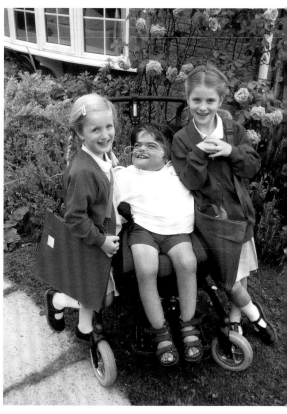

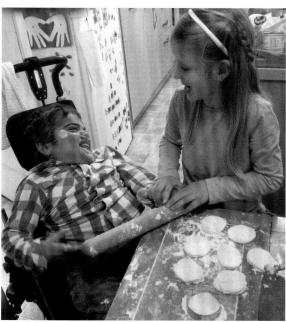

Left: Baking with my Susannah.

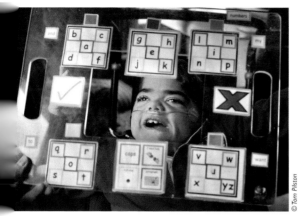

Left: With my spelling board.

Right: A selection of nouns on my writing word board.

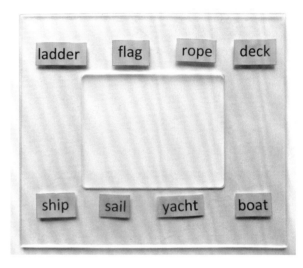

ladder	flag	rope	deck
ship	sail	yacht	boat

question word		Verb
superlative	negative	
		adverb
adjective		
preposition	noun	abc
	connective	

Left: My writing board.

Right: Meeting Edward
Timpson, who was at
the time the Minister
of State for Vulnerable
Children and Families.

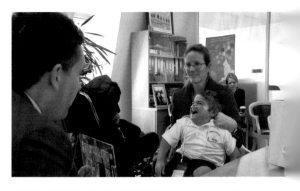

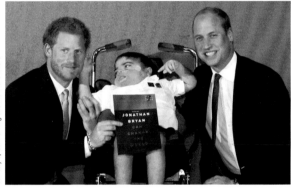

Left: Receiving a
Diana Legacy Award
from Prince William
and Prince Harry.

Below: Mummy
delivering my speech
at a reception at the
House of Lords.

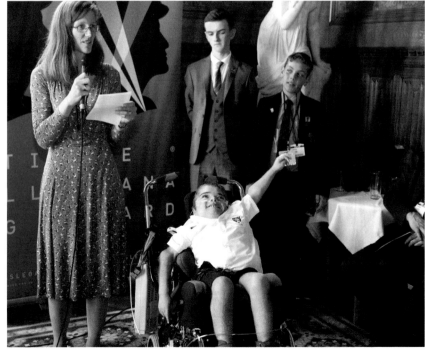

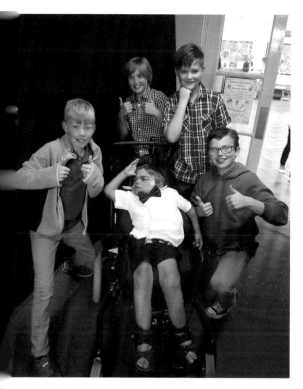

Left: At the premiere of the CBBC *My Life* programme with my primary school friends.

Below: Two writers meeting – Sir Michael Morpurgo and me.

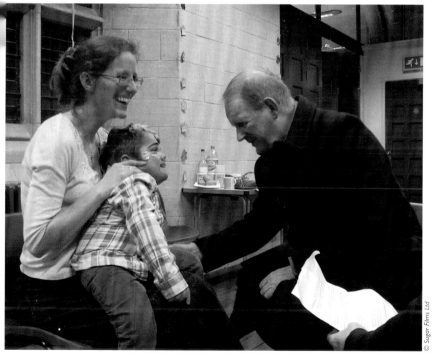

© Sugar Films Ltd

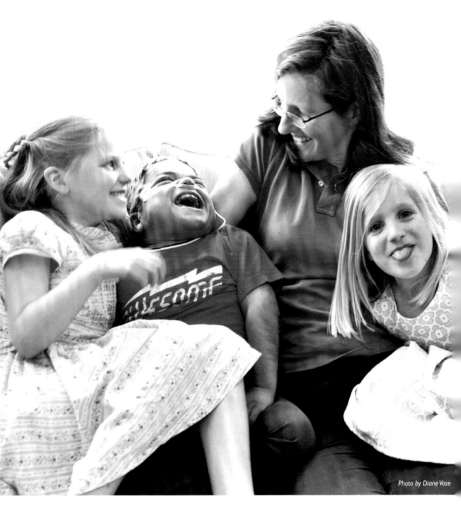

Photo by Diane Vose

Surrounded by my favourite girls.

crew. Annoyingly, my teacher Sarah was making me write a story map. In a bid to make this activity more 'fun', the plan was disguised as a mountain. Not a small hill, but a steep, craggy mountain struggling to be constrained within an A3 piece of paper. Every face of this edifice needed filling in with the tedious detail of each scene, while the story was bursting to be let out of the confines of my brain. For each word I wrote, a selection of options had been Blu-Tacked to a Perspex board; I needed to demonstrate I had read every word before settling my gaze on the one I wanted. Hundreds of small pieces of card, each featuring a single word, were kept in a large folder which was parked next to the desk, black and brooding like a dark cloud waiting to shower its words on the page. Scaling this mountain was painstakingly slow torture; choosing each word was so frustrating when the adventure was desperate to set sail.

During the week my story plan was making painful progress, making the weekend all the more full of escape. And this weekend was extra-special because it was my Jemima's birthday. Of the things I love in life, holidays and birthdays are near the top.

Every holiday we escape landlocked Wiltshire for the seaside, exchanging views of rolling fields hemmed in dark green for the wide, wild vistas of the ocean. This holiday was no different. On the beach, we were all overcome with the moment: the wide expanse of deserted sand, the ocean rollers beating the shore and dragging it back. Propelled in my chair, we broke into a jubilant run. With the sea air filling my worn-out lungs, and the cold January wind whipping my face, I felt the exhilaration of being alive. Alive to celebrate Jemima turning three. Alive to enjoy my family on another holiday. Alive to breathe in the beauty of creation. But my voice was locked inside my alive brain.

Travelling the narrow north Devon sunken lanes framed by van-high hedges, we crawled our way to a small secluded pub in a village by a bay. Cocooned inside the wood-panelled room, the fire emitting its warming glow, we shed our outer layers of coats, scarves, gloves, hats and jumpers until we were each surrounded by strata of clothing, littered around us like the discarded leaves of a cabbage. Looking around the table I gazed at the shiny windswept faces of those I love the most, and my heart was full of contented gratitude. But as the candles were stuck into Jemima's pudding and we all sang for her, this moment was fringed with sadness that I couldn't join my voice to the family chorus telling her how much we loved her.

When we came back from our holiday I returned to my story map, refreshed and with renewed energy and enthusiasm. To my delight Sarah said I could get on with my story. At last. Having spent interminable hours envisioning the opening scene, I could now, finally, put it onto paper. The process was still painstakingly slow. The clear board, which Mummy called my writing board, with pieces of coloured paper stuck on it was held in front of me, each colour denoting a different part of speech. Green for verbs, yellow for nouns, bright-blue for adverbs, grey for adjectives, brown for question words, lilac for prepositions, white for connectives and conjunctions and a little square with 'abc', which transported me to the spelling board. Once I had chosen a colour, Sarah and Mummy sprang into action, selecting words for me to choose from. Rifling through the folder, Sarah and Mummy muttered to each other.

'Oh yes, that's a great one.'

'What about this word? Or do you think it's too like that word?'

Conversations about words filled the air for minutes at a time while I waited. Finally, the 'great word', the 'word like that word' and the 'try that one' word, along with many others, were held in front of me – Blu-Tacked to the Perspex board, while Sarah pointed to each word in turn, making sure I had read them all before I fixed my gaze on the chosen one. Chosen from words selected for me. Not words I would necessarily write... if I could. Slow would be an understatement, as my story was meticulously pieced together; each word taking two Perspex boards (a writing board and a word board), a large file of possible words, hours of preparation, and Blu-Tack as a regular grocery item. And all the time, the precise word I wanted was invariably not there and I was reduced to asking them questions in my head. Frustration sometimes got the better of me, as I deleted the whole morning's sentence with repeated looks at the delete sign. Irritation was thus shared with those supporting me. Unfortunately, frustration shared is not frustration halved; and with exasperation electrifying both sides of the board, we started again.

While in English I made sluggish progress, maths became my light relief; numbers and patterns had always attracted me, and now they combined in a lesson on prediction.

As a sheet of small circular stickers with pictures of cartoon faces on was waved in front of me, I was asked to predict the total number of stickers. Looking at the number board ahead of me, I stared at the 1 then the 8 before smiling, my signal to Sarah on the other side of the board that 18 was my answer. Pause. Mummy was now taking twice as long as me to count the stickers. Pause.

'Did you know the total was 18, or did you make a lucky guess?' said Mummy, looking at me in bewilderment.

'How did you know the answer when you hadn't had time to count them?' asked Sarah.

It was her turn to be astounded. Confounded, even.

By the time Sarah and Mummy had gathered enough composure to show me a further three sheets of stickers, I just needed to glance at them to make sure they had the same pattern as the previous sheets, before looking at the 5 then the 4.

'How are you doing this, Jonathan?' Sarah and Mummy chorused, with a mixture of astonishment and pride.

I couldn't tell them. I had no voice.

The following morning, eager to see if yesterday's lesson was a fluke, Sarah and Mummy forwent their usual ritual of morning pleasantries, as Sarah produced from her bag some robot wrapping paper for me to look at. As usual, they gave me three seconds to take in the detail. Clearly there were nine robots in three lines, so 27 in all. Pause. Mummy was counting again.

'There's only 26. One of the robots in the middle line is missing,' she said slowly.

Bother. I hate getting things wrong.

Strangely, this didn't dampen their bewilderment; undeterred, they fetched the Lego bricks from the cupboard. First, one brick was fastened to the baseplate – it had four studs. Next, five bricks were added, and with nothing missing, I found the total number of studs easy to calculate. Rows of bricks mounted up in pleasing patterns, two rows of red, two rows of yellow; each time I accurately indicated the answer on my maths board. Finally, Mummy sniggered as she added a single line of three blue bricks. Nice try. Looking at the numbers in front of me, I told her the answer was 60.

'Nearly, Jonathan. The answer is... 62.' There was a degree of satisfaction in Mummy's voice. Finding out her son wasn't a mathematical genius was obviously the cause of some relief.

'Jonathan is right, Chantal. The answer is 60,' Sarah whispered. After over a year of increasingly difficult addition and subtraction in home school maths lessons, this was a moment of enlightenment for them. As the colour drained from Mummy's face, Sarah was sent to unearth Daddy from his sabbatical study.

While my mother has sat for hour upon hour of home school, my father's main involvement has been the welcome interruptions of morning coffee. With the mindset of a scientist, he has also been my most sceptical supporter. All the time Mummy eulogised about what I was achieving, Daddy would be the voice of rational reasoning. As a result, he had observed me answering questions about books I had read, doing spelling tests with different carers holding my spelling board, and watched Mummy closing her eyes to prove she wasn't moving my head.

Entering the room with disbelief etched in his smile, Daddy listened and scrutinised as the methodology was explained. With the baseboard in hand, he started rearranging the squares of

Lego into random patterns, taking some off and adding others. The final product was presented to me for the customary three seconds... Tension hung in the concentration. Like an external examiner, Daddy declared time was up; sidling to behind the number board, he watched as I looked at the 5 then the 6. Pause.

'Is he right?' Mummy had obviously not had the minutes she would need to complete the task, and Sarah had not seen the question, but Daddy's maths is good.

'I have no idea,' exclaimed Daddy, taking the baseboard and counting each square of four. '14 times four is 56.' Incredulity wiped out scepticism, as Daddy's jaw momentarily dropped. 'How do you do this, Jonathan?' Daddy seemed genuinely perplexed.

It was my turn to be confounded when Mummy made a pattern for him, and he couldn't tell us the number of studs in three seconds. But my father knows everything! If only I could ask him, 'How can you *not* do it?'

Thus followed a series of mental maths

challenges, whereby I was verbally asked: 7 lots of 8, 9 groups of 15, 20 lots of 18. Why did Mummy and Sarah always check my answers on the calculator? And why was it so funny when I got it right? Apparently, there is even a symbol for this – 'x'. It's called multiplication.

But I was reduced to asking them these questions in my head. For while I could easily use my number board, my spelling board was only used for my daily spelling test and as a little 'abc' option on my writing board. Before breakfast every morning, we started playing a game where I was given a word to spell on my spelling board: Mummy's idea to help me learn the placing of letters on the spelling board. Navigating around my spelling board took time. If only the alphabet was made up of just ten digits like my number board! With so many letters, I needed to remember where each one was located, what colour it was, and where the colours were placed.

This is how the spelling board works:

The 26 letters of the alphabet are organised into

5 grids of letters, and each letter is surrounded by one of five colours – blue, red, green, yellow or purple. To select a letter, I needed to move my eyes twice across the board – to a group of letters and to the corresponding coloured square. For example, if I want to say 'Hi,' I look at the grid the 'h' is in, and because the 'h' is green, I then look at the green square. Next I look at the grid the 'i' is in, and because the 'i' is red, I then look at the red square. My communication partner points where I am looking, and sounds out the letters. Bottom middle is my space bar, and the tick and cross are my 'yes' and 'no', with the cross doubling up as a delete function.

With five carers and Sarah and Mummy as communication partners, there were eight of us learning how the spelling board worked! In my wheelchair I find it slower; as my head moves around, carers have to dance with me, following the movements of my head with the spelling board. In busy environments I can't resist the temptation to see what is going on, resulting in less spelling and more dancing. But Mummy is the ultimate in comfortable seating; while on her knee, I am at my optimal spelling speed.

During my writing time, it was a daily toss-up between the frustratingly limited word options I was presented with on the writing board — vocabulary limited to words used by seven year olds — and the slow, complicated precision required by my spelling board. With my intense dislike of getting anything wrong, I was not ready to use the spelling board for more than an occasional word at a time.

Gradually, as time progressed, the satisfaction of spelling out the exact word I wanted to use outweighed all the other factors: my writing board's laborious system that only offered pre-chosen words, the exactitude required by the spelling board and the time it took to construct each word. Above all I am a perfectionist, and the spelling board was my gateway to the perfect word fit.

Meanwhile I continued my story with Alexander, 'Egged On'. So far Alexander and Jonathan had endured a dangerous sea crossing to capture some enemy eggs. Today, I had a particular word in mind for my story. A descriptive word, a sonorous word. The perfect word.

For as long as I could remember, Mummy had read to me: Bible stories, funny stories, short stories, *The Chronicles of Narnia*. For days, weeks and months we had curled up in a hospital bed together and plunged ourselves into a novel. Immersing myself in a story is the most enjoyable, wonderful escapism; books have nourished my mind and prevented mental decay during my years of silence. Trapped in cerebral palsy I run within the pages: skipping, laughing, exploring. Plunging myself into the adventure of new tales, I have inhabited the scenes of authors' pictures and woven them with my imagination. Words have been my portal to another world. And now the mantle was passing on to me.

During the nine years of being effectively locked in by my severe cerebral palsy, words and phrases had been banked while my mother read to me. Unable to develop the physical skills of my peers, maybe my mind had more room for academic learning.

Picking up the spelling board, Sarah's finger pointed to where my eyes were looking. Sitting on Mummy's lap, our bodies remained still as Sarah's finger danced to the rhythm of my eyes. Following my lead, we slow-waltzed around the board, synchronised to the music of the word in my head. At first we were like clumsy teenagers trying to learn — stumbling, slow and stilted.

'Jonathan, today you've written: "Tired from slaying the ships enemies they towed" — what do you want to write next?' Mummy enquired. She had already been surprised by the word 'slaying', as it wasn't even an option in the verb section of the big black folder.

As the duet continued I spelt out an 'm' then a 'y'. Because the process was so exacting and tiring, and because I wanted to draw out the suspense, I closed my eyes. After the usual cajoling to open them, I started to enjoy the ensuing conversation:

'Did he put a space after the "y"?' Mummy needed to know, as she was also typing what I wrote into the computer.

'He hasn't yet, but I expect he will when he opens up again. I can't think what else he would want to write beginning "my".' Sarah obviously had no idea of the word I was crafting. Before they started chatting again about the fate of the near obsolete folder that brimmed with many hours of their dedicated input, I opened up — ready for play to recommence.

'My... "r"... "i"... "a"... "d"... "s".' Mummy articulated each letter of the word rally, but Sarah was so engrossed in mirroring my eyes with her finger she had lost the word.

'Myriads.' Mummy looked at Sarah, who stared back at her, stunned.

Their silence heralded the beginning of the end of mine.

It took Mummy one more day to realise that now I could spell everything I wanted to write, I could also spell everything I wanted to say.

Now it was my turn to be the custodian of the power of words. My challenge to capture delicately the image and bequeath it words that let it breathe. Like a bird let out of its cage, the picture that words can generate was free to fly in my reader's mind and assume a new life of its own.

CHAPTER FIVE

A Family of Haikus

Imaginative
playmate, soulmate, laughing fun –
Pretty Susannah!

Unconditional
loving, singing, full of joy –
Cuddly Jemima!

Intellectual
mantime, cavetime, piece of quiet –
Faithfully Daddy!

Incomparable
mother, teacher, one with me –
Devoted Mummy!

WHAT DO YOU ASK YOUR NINE-YEAR-OLD CHILD, WHO CAN NOW TELL YOU ANYTHING? No need to predict what he wants, no need to try and interpret his smiles for pre-set answers — he can just spell it out for himself. Anything I asked, Jonathan could tell me. As I sat supporting his body on my lap in our playroom, with the girls running in and out, and Christopher cooking in the kitchen, I wondered where to start. Sat opposite us was a carer, spelling board poised — expectant, waiting. Now that Jonathan, the carers, Sarah and I had learnt how to use the board, after nine years of silence, so many of my questions had evaporated into the mists of time, and all I could think of were questions I already knew the answer to.

'What is your favourite ice-cream?'

'Choc.' The spelling was still slow and deliberate.

'Chocolate. We knew that already, Mummy. Why don't you ask him a question we don't know?' Susannah interjected before skipping out of the room to continue her game with Jemima.

'I know, Jonathan, how about this one. What

is your earliest memory?' Again, I felt I probably knew the answer, but I couldn't be sure.

'Susannah out of you,' Jonathan replied.

(Transcripts of this conversation and others like it read now like someone who is learning a foreign language, where the meaning of the words is present, but the syntax isn't quite right. A child's attempts at conversation from the land of silence.)

Ever the diplomat, Jonathan evened this out by answering the next question (what did he remember about our previous home?) with a mention of not having 'kind sister Jemima'. In the very early stages of my pregnancy with Jemima, Jonathan had once again been very ill, and so – partly as an incentive to him to pull through, and partly because if he didn't, I wanted him to know about her, even if he never got to meet her – she had become our shared whispered secret. When the secret became a real baby sister, he was as delighted with her as he had been with Susannah. In the early months Jemima and Jonathan would often fall asleep together, with Jemima lying on him, or next to him, but usually with their faces turned towards each other.

General memories seemed a good line of questioning for Jonathan. What he could remember from his early life was illuminating in showing how his past experiences had shaped the present.

'What can you remember about being in hospital, Jonathan?'

'I have to get better,' he spelled out.

'What did he say?' It was hard for Christopher to follow the conversation from the other room, above the noise of sausages spitting in the pan. 'I know.' Daddy's turn for a question now. 'How did you feel in hospital?'

'Ill,' was the response.

We all laughed, as Jonathan managed to convey in a single word that silly questions get silly answers. Acutely aware that the phrasing of the questions was important, I knew it was crucial not to lead him to certain answers. After essentially being restricted to yes or no answers all his life, I now wanted to encourage as broad an answer as I could.

'What is important to you?'

'Mummy, Jesus, Susannah, Jemima, Daddy, sisters.'

Like a walk with many paths, we were experimenting, going down different avenues to see where it would take us and what the view looked like.

'Jesus?' I asked. After all, he had been surrounded by Christians all of his life.

'S… e… e… n.' Jonathan spelled out.

'Seen. What have you seen?'

Like the atmosphere before the curtain draws back for a play, there was an intensity in waiting to hear what he would write next. Suddenly this had transformed from a chit-chat to something more profound, and the atmosphere reflected it.

'His house.'

'When did you see his house, Jonathan?' My voice trembled. What did this mean? What was he talking about?

'Small, most meet me is when my in pain. His men met my parents. My racing, I up trees.'

Opposite me the carer who had been with us for

many years, through hospital stays and intensive care admissions, sat with shining eyes, and although it was warm, I could see the hairs on her arm were standing up. As the conversation was relayed between the kitchen and the playroom, and again to the girls, we all spent our supper time trying to understand what Jonathan could mean, while he sat beside us, beaming a smile of relief. A smile of, 'I've wanted to tell you this for so long...'

During the following months, this was a topic of conversation that we would revisit, carefully, as if it was a fragile, precious experience that we mustn't handle too clumsily, for fear we could impose our growing understanding on it.

Other questions we asked didn't get the answer we expected. When Jonathan started to be able to talk to us, I assumed, like most people, that it must have been the most frustrating thing to have been unable to tell people what he wanted. Although Jonathan didn't seem frustrated, I imagined that he hid it well beneath a veneer of contentment. One day we were in the kitchen at breakfast time, and as usual I had got him ready for the day ahead. What frustrated Jonathan most?

'Having my face washed,' he spelled out, and gave me an award-winning grin.

Typical boy!

When Jonathan began using the spelling board, our family relationships shifted and altered; at home it was his time with Christopher that changed the most. Silence has always characterised the time that Christopher and Jonathan spend together – silence, it seems, is a very necessary component of 'man time', so even now that they could have a conversation it didn't seem on the outside to change much. But Christopher has an academic's instincts, and now they shared time with each other more as equals, looking things up together, discussing what they had found out.

Now we had a child who could ask for anything he wanted. One such conversation sticks in the mind.

From the week before Susannah was born we have had day carers to help me, paid for by the insurance award from the car accident; an extra pair of hands to help with three small children and all the equipment and extra needs that Jonathan has. Much of what Jonathan has achieved would not have been possible without these carers working hard behind the scenes – making up feeds, medicines, filling up oxygen tanks and accompanying Jonathan to school. They have all mastered the spelling board. Night carers have helped me to sleep, so essential for functioning well in the day. Claire has been with us from the beginning, and even brought in her tiny baby to meet him. This fragile baby looked far too small to endure one of Jonathan's spasms, so, although he loves babies, I said that he couldn't hold him, as his sisters manoeuvred themselves onto the sofa to receive the tiny bundle. Spelling was a relatively new skill for Jonathan, so, keen to have a chat with his carer, we got the board.

After a few pleasantries, Jonathan said, 'I need a brother.'

Having gone to the effort of spelling it out, letter by letter, surely Mummy would now give him what he wanted!

As the new mother left, Jonathan moved onto Daddy with his question, along with his solution to the fact that we were not considering having another child: 'Foster.' Still not taking no for an answer, he turned to his carer on the other side of the spelling board. What he didn't know was that she had mentioned to me that she was very unlikely to be able to have children of her own.

'Pippa have one,' spelled out Jonathan.

Nervous laughter from Pippa the carer; embarrassed closing-the-subject chatter from us. A year later Pippa asked me into our sitting room for a meeting...

She was pregnant.

Over the following months we started slowly to ask Jonathan more questions, always trying to be careful never to ask leading questions, but keen to understand what we could. It takes a lot to make me speechless, but many times I have been left without words. One day he gave a detailed description of the moment we had intercepted a police car on our way to Bristol when he collapsed on dialysis – specifying where Christopher and

I were, and what was happening. But it was his description of his time in the garden that blew us away the most.

Chantal Bryan

CHAPTER SIX

Baking Beauty

Filling, beating, stirring, pouring,
Baking beauty life restoring,
Dripping goodness love in sharing,
Aromatic health repairing,
Pleasant parcels held with pleasure,
Tantalising tastes to treasure.

AT LAST, I COULD TELL MY FAMILY ABOUT MY TIME IN THE GARDEN. At last. This was the one early memory Mummy knew nothing about. For nine years she had shared every aspect of my life; when I was admitted to hospital, she effectively became an inpatient with me, only leaving our bed to go and get some food. At home, when I wanted to play, she sat behind me supporting my body and helping my hands to manipulate the toys. If I was tired, she read to me; if I was excited, we played instruments; if we needed some fresh air, she took me into the garden or for a walk. During playdates, while other mummies chatted and drank coffee, my mummy carried me through the soft play area so I could keep up with my friends. If I went out to a group, she had to go with me. But I had visited the garden on my own. My most significant, wonderful memory had never been shared until now.

Describing what is beyond description is almost impossible. How I got there? I do not remember. However, my memory of my time there is as crystal clear as if I had visited yesterday.

Since sharing this part of my story, my parents have been helping me understand the events around my experience. When an intensive care consultant tells you that your child is being put into an induced coma in order for the ventilator to work as best it can, you know it is serious. But when you enter intensive care and find every consultant and doctor on the ward in your child's room telling you that it could go either way, you know this could be it. While my body hung in the balance, I was already tasting what it was like on the other side.

Alive. I had never felt so alive. Free from my crippled, dysfunctional body, I ran. Ran! Fresh, verdant grass beneath my supple feet. A warm, soft breeze caressed my face. Sounds of children's laughter mingled with birdsong. Freedom!

For the first time, I could see clearly — like the murkiness had been blown away to reveal abundant meadows of spring flowers swaying their heads under the mellow sunlight. As I stretched my body to its full height (my scoliosis had elongated and vanished altogether), I realised the dragon cerebral palsy had been banished from the lair of my body. All my life this monster had subjugated my body to painful spasms, distorting and writhing my frame, breathing fire under my skin, stealing my voice; and now it was dead and defeated forever! With the sibilance of my oxygen silenced, I inhaled deeply, the fresh air vitalising my new body and filling my soul with joy. Swinging my free arms, I sauntered through an orchard; the trees, laden with delectable fruit, stretched beckoning branches towards me. Savouring every moment, enjoying the harmony between my perfect, new body and my soul, I was whole. Groups of children were playing near the trees, their mellifluous voices drawing me closer. Happiness was not merely a facial expression for the people I met; joy exuded from them, and the atmosphere was saturated in a deep, contented peace. As I neared them, I wanted to ask where I was. And I could! I just thought it and spoke.

'Jesus' garden.' The melodic reply danced in my soul.

And that's when I saw him: Noah, my beautiful

friend who had died the year before from a brain tumour. Although Noah was a few years younger than me, I had cuddled him as a baby and played with him as a toddler, at his house, at my house and in church. Adored by those who knew him and treasured by his young mother, his sudden illness and rapid decline had shaken our community and devastated his family. Capturing in words those moments of reunion is so hard, but as the time drew on, I was aware that I had a choice to make. Either I could stay to meet the gardener, my author, my saviour; or I could go back. Back to my fragile, sick body; back to my mind trapped in my silence; back to the family I loved.

'Jonathan.' My mother's voice called me from beyond the garden, and my decision was made. That decision was the hardest of my life, but it has also shaped my perspective on life since. While my soul longs to live in the garden forever, my heart is torn between my family and the garden, but with Jesus' presence helping me here, I know I can endure my limiting body for longer. My experience in the garden has given me a zest for life here and a zeal for life there.

While I am still trapped in my body here I want to be involved in decisions about it. Before the days of my spelling board, every time we went to clinic, Mummy would talk to the doctors about me; what was wrong with me, courses of treatment and plans for the future. Between Dr Dudley and Mummy there is an encyclopaedic knowledge of my past and present medical history — I sometimes imagine a gameshow with them pitted against each other on the specialist subject, 'Jonathan Bryan'. It is a very close contest!

Together Dr Dudley and my parents have inhabited some difficult places, and navigated some tricky paths, holding and balancing my quality of life and my prognosis. Now I can ask the questions directly. My favourite questions now in the various clinics I attend are: 'Will I get better?' and 'How long have I got?' Some consultants find the questions from the child in the wheelchair a bit disarming, but I enjoy watching their barely disguised shock and listening to their measured responses.

Most of all, I can now add my voice to plans for the future, and when I talk, people seem to listen. So, I have told medical professionals how I want to go and where I want to be; for while going is exciting for me, how I get there is not something I look forward to. Meeting with the palliative care consultant, I have also chatted about what a worn-out body looks and feels like. Apparently, most people find that food is not important to them at the end, but I made sure it was given a top priority in my plan. At the end of the day, I am still a hungry 12-year-old boy!

All my life, people have done things for me. I am washed, dressed, fed via a tube and wheeled around. Now I have found my voice, I want to use it to help other people. Before I could talk, Mummy would have listed baking as one of the things I liked doing occasionally. She was in for a shock.

'I want to bake every day.' Sometimes using my spelling board is so satisfying.

'That's nice, darling.' Mummy was enjoying our conversations as much as me. 'Every day for a week?'

Frowning, I looked at the 'no' sign.

'Every day for a month?' Mummy's voice was rising in panic; baking takes time and energy, and with three small children, time and energy are in short supply.

'Every day forever.'

Thus started a chain of events that led to me getting a bread maker for my birthday. My best present ever.

Home baking has the power to make people extraordinarily happy. And now my baking can spread that joy too. While I still need help to weigh the ingredients, and many kitchen tasks need to be performed with Mummy's hand over mine, I can now use my spelling board to direct how much goes in and when. Sometimes you hit on a recipe that becomes your baking signature. Mine is brownies.

Jonathan's Brownies

These chocolate brownies have become known as 'Jonathan's brownies'. I didn't invent the recipe but I have made them for family, friends and as presents for teachers more than any other recipe. With a delicious melt-in-the-mouth richness, some people who know me are prepared to buy this book for the brownie recipe alone! My sisters say they can taste the love with which I make them.

Ingredients
10 oz / 275g butter
13 oz / 375g caster sugar *
4 eggs
1 tsp baking powder
3 oz / 75g cocoa *
4 oz / 100g plain flour
1 packet of cooking chocolate drops *

* *These ingredients could be Fairtrade, something I am passionate about supporting.*

Method

- Line a deep-sided, well-greased roasting tin with baking parchment, and pre-heat the oven to gas mark 3 / 160°C / fan 140°C.

- Cream the butter and sugar in the food processor.

- Add all the rest of the ingredients except the chocolate drops into the processor and mix well.

- Remove the blade and stir in the chocolate drops.

- Spoon the mixture into the roasting tin.

- Bake at gas mark 3 / 160°C / fan 140°C for about 12 minutes, making sure that the mixture doesn't burn.

- Turn the heat down to gas mark 1 / 140°C / fan 120°C for about another 40 minutes until the top of the cake no longer wobbles, and a skewer comes out clean.

- Cut into pieces while warm, leave to cool before taking out.

Although I can't eat the final products, the aroma of my brownies fills the kitchen, the house and my nose until I can almost taste them. But my greatest pleasure comes from giving them away and watching people's expressions as they devour them, savouring every last crumb.

As well as baking, my spelling board gives me the freedom to tell my family about more surprising things I want to do. Perhaps one of the most unexpected things I have always wished to play with is Lego. Utilising my board, I can now not just ask for Lego, I can say what I want to construct and how. Lego has also given me a gateway to interact with my friends and we have even made stop-motion movie clips using the iPad.

Ever since I was four, I had been going to my local primary school for one afternoon a week, joining my peers for the afternoon session and attending the lesson with them. Despite a common belief about the indiscriminate blind acceptance of children, in my experience both children and adults can be divided: those who can connect with me, and those who can't see past the physical barriers. Thankfully, I was blessed with solid, dependable friends at my primary school who connected with me and included me in their games. For them, my new way to spell everything I wanted to say was just another way for us to communicate; one method among many. We still went around the playground together, still had our secrets, still enjoyed each other's company. Through my years of silence those friends had been my loyal companions; steady, true comrades through the maze of growing up.

However, for the other children my new ability brought a dramatic change of attitude in the classroom, because now I could join in. When I was part of a small group discussion, I was no longer the silent onlooker; when the class were asked a question, I now had a chance to contribute my answer. And friends at my primary school were getting good at using my spelling board. Now they could all pick it up for a quick yes or no answer from me, and one friend, Rochelle, even studied how my carers used it so that she could see what I was spelling. After a month of observing the spelling system, she became a communication partner too. At last I could chat to my friends without grown-ups around. Now I was not just chronologically in Year 4; I was academically in Year 4.

Before, it didn't matter what lessons I joined my peers for, as the main purpose was always social interaction with children my own age. However, now I could communicate well and prove my learning, Mummy and Daddy asked the local school to consider increasing my time there from one to two afternoons a week. And they said yes! Not only that, but the teacher even moved the subjects around so that I could attend the more academic sessions.

If only we had felt that same level of jubilation at my special school. Or witnessed a fraction of the excitement. Or even a 'Well done.' Instead, everything continued in much the same way as it always had. Most frustratingly of all, it seemed to us that no one, except the one-to-one teaching assistant (TA) assigned to me, believed that I could spell using the alphabet board. Apparently it was less challenging for the special school to think that my mother, my five carers, Sarah (a primary school teacher), and their own employed TA were kidding themselves, than it was to explore the implications for me and the other eight children in the class, or indeed all the children who are mislabelled with profound and multiple learning difficulties.

When I looked at my friend Will, my heart was filled with a deep sadness; he had always been my special school academic partner, often overtaking me in his demonstrated learning; for his eye-pointing has been consistently clearer than mine. But now there was no satisfaction in being the first, no gratification in the top position, because suddenly, seemingly overnight, I had gone into a league of my own. On my own. Alone. And it was lonely and depressing watching the isolation of my friends, who had no independent way to communicate.

Instead they were mostly relying on facial

expressions to make choices, either smiling as they heard the option they wanted, or choosing between two objects placed in front of them. Prior to spelling, my communication had been limited to this too. Before my eyes were discovered as the only part of my body that I could control, my private speech and language therapist set up a communication file for me to use. Everything in the file was categorised, and I had to smile as the category I wanted was read out. Smiling is not as quick or easy for me to control as my eyes; it takes effort and time and is unreliable. On average it took four smiles to arrive at a word. And often the exact word wasn't there. And there were some things I didn't feel like smiling for – for example, who wants to smile to say they have a headache? It was slow and so boring that after a certain number of smiles I gave up, even if I hadn't chosen any words. But in its defence, at least someone was really trying to present me with the option of a bank of words I could choose from.

The key for me, and children like me, is to find out what we can independently control, and then use this as our access to the curriculum. I never had profound and multiple learning difficulties, but I did have profound and multiple difficulties in accessing learning. It should be that there is an expectation for all children to learn, regardless of their physical disability or label. When my access was in its infancy, numerous pieces of equipment and techniques were used, but when my eyes were my access, there was one machine which held out some hope for me — the eye-gaze machine. Patiently my private speech and language therapist tried out different models of eye-gaze machine with me, and eventually we seemed to find one that worked. But it was slow and inaccurate compared to my spelling board. Frustratingly inaccurate. In the end I suggested we chuck the eye-gaze machine out of the window.

Around this time Will got his own eye-gaze machine, but rather than seeing this as the beginning of an exciting communication and learning journey, it was viewed as the end. With an eye-gaze machine Will could choose from an array of pre-determined options with a picture and word underneath, rather like my communication file. For example, in the 'feelings' section of my file, I could choose 'sad', 'bored' or 'angry', but not 'frustrated', which is what using the file made me feel. If no one taught Will to read and write he would be stuck with those options – unless he was so intelligent that he could teach himself to read and write from the words under the pictures. You don't suddenly start using an alphabet board – you have to be taught how to read and write first. Being able to spell words gives you the freedom to say exactly what you want. If special school takes the decision not to teach you to read and write, who will?

Meanwhile, my home education had morphed into a test centre. Unusually, for a child of my age, I love tests, particularly tests I need to think about a bit, and enjoy working out the answer. Before I started using the spelling board and my ability with numbers came to light, Sarah and Mummy were following a Year I syllabus; now they were trying to work out what academic year to teach me. Helpfully for me, the government set tests for the end of Year 2, and I had devoured them, getting good percentages. However, rather than move on to the Year 3 syllabus, it was decided that I should sit some Year 3 papers – but the novelty of tests was waning. Half a term later, I was sitting Year 4 exams, and not only had the initial excitement worn off completely, but I was increasingly irritated by the maths questions I couldn't do, because I hadn't covered the syllabus.

Armed with the marked papers for Year 4, Mummy went to visit the head of the special school. Surely now the significance of what had happened to me would penetrate the system?

'These are impressive test results,' concluded the head, 'but until we see Jonathan use the board in school, we can't do anything about it.'

Concurrently, I was in the corridor outside the office spelling to my school-employed teaching assistant, 'My mother is seeing the head.'

While we felt that the special school was fundamentally not interested, numerous people in the communities I am part of became fascinated with my new abilities. One of them, an educational psychologist, volunteered her skills and arrived with the ultimate entertaining test: a cognitive assessment which Mummy told me was rather like an IQ test. Sitting on Mummy's knee, I was presented with a line diagram, and after a few seconds the page was turned to reveal more line drawings, but only one was the same as on the previous page. Each option corresponded to a square on a Perspex board which I used to indicate my answer. Blessed with a photographic memory, I found the test an exciting challenge, and as it progressed in difficulty I started to get more right than Mummy, who would give her answer after I'd given mine.

'And that's the end of the test.' The educational psychologist had a look of shocked amazement, but we had little idea as to the significance.

'What age do the tests go up to?' Mummy enquired.

'This test is used for children up to the age of 18. I stop the test when the person taking it gets more than five wrong in each section. It is not often I finish the test.'

The results of this test were verified by the local council, who sent their own educational psychologist to do a different cognitive assessment. She reported that I scored on the 99th percentile for a child my age.

Following the tests, Mummy once again phoned various members of the extended family. I suspect by now they were getting used to conversations detailing my latest achievements. Reactions from those not in my immediate family were split into those who found it 'unbelievable', and those who 'knew all along' that my mind worked. Mostly, those in the latter category were people who have spent hours with me, often alone. But now I can join in. So when Gran plays a crossword game I can give my 'penny's worth', and when she plays cribbage I am no longer the silent onlooker but a fiercely competitive player.

When we lived in our previous parish, a recently retired teacher took me out in my wheelchair to visit anyone who was old and lonely. Sitting on their doorstep, I would wave and smile and make their day a little brighter, before we moved on to the next house. I see this as a special God-given way I could give happiness back, enabled by a lady who always believed I was in there, always knew I understood and always loved me as I was.

Then there was my granny. Like the fifth emergency service, Grannie always had her little red suitcase packed and ready at the door. Prepared for every eventuality, her case filled with identical sets of navy-blue skirts and checked shirts, Grannie would arrive with willing hands for Mummy and Daddy and a warm, comforting cuddle for me. Long, glorious hours were spent nestling in my Grannie's arms, enclosed in her loving acceptance. She was 'not in the least bit surprised' when I learnt to communicate using my spelling board, and as I've explained neither was almost anyone else who had spent large amounts of time with me.

However, there was one notable exception to this rule: Grandpa. At six foot three, Grandpa's large presence and personality fill the room; his deep voice resonates, satiating the atmosphere with gravitas. Never having encountered disability in his youth, Grandpa is scared, almost phobic, of it; so while I have never doubted his love for me, he has visibly struggled with my physical limitations, which had formed an impenetrable barrier to him getting to know me. Until now.

Before, when he met me, he would wave his hand vigorously in front of me, like a windscreen wiper, and say loudly and clearly, 'Hello Jonathan,' before turning to Mummy and asking, 'He can hear me, can he darling?'

The irony is he's quite deaf, and my hearing is better than his. Once I began to spell he was blown away by the abilities of his grandson, who he had previously thought of as unable to do anything. Even so, it took him a little while to adjust to the fact that I now spelt everything. So when he tried to disguise my birthday surprise by spelling it out to Mummy, I was laughing before she had even worked out the word.

As a linguist, Grandpa loves words, and now we can discuss them together, luxuriating in their diversity and richness, jointly finding the perfect match. For Grandpa, my use of a spelling board has been an epiphanic moment, and his company has become among the most stimulating for me.

Many people assume that the best thing about my spelling board is being able to chat, but for me, creative writing will always be my first love.

CHAPTER SEVEN

Holidays

Happiness emerging, excitement growing,
Oceans of dancing waves lovingly flowing,
Laughter like singing birds heard in the morning,
Irresistible ice-cream, noon-time yawning,
Daddy filling our heads with figures and facts,
Away we're escaping down unexplored tracks,
Yearly adventures treasured deep in our hearts,
Sadness it's over 'til the next one starts.

WHILE THE SPECIAL SCHOOL NEVER SEEMED TO BELIEVE ME, THE LOCAL VILLAGE PRIMARY SCHOOL EMBRACED MY NEW WAY TO COMMUNICATE, NEVER DOUBTING MY ABILITIES, AND THEY TRANSLATED THIS INTO A PLACE ON THEIR REGISTER. As a fully fledged member of the class they took my desire to learn as seriously as they had taken my need for social interaction. During the mornings at home I would follow the English and maths curriculum that they were doing at school, but at the optimal speed I could manage in my own environment; with one, sometimes two people as board holders and scribes. And Mummy as the ultimate in comfortable, adaptable seating.

After I became unlocked, the words, images and feelings that filled my head became a bubbling mass looking for ways to be expressed. Being a pupil at mainstream primary school gave me the literary tools and instruction I needed, introducing me to different genres and techniques so that my emergent creative writing could flourish. So I started to embark on writing a 500-word story for a BBC Radio 2 competition and to learn how to shape language for different purposes. In all the subjects I was soaking up the new learning, but it wasn't just the learning I was included in.

The residential. Like a rite of passage, all Year 5s and 6s go on residential each year, and when I say all I mean *all*. Including me! When I was on the register of my special school, my class went away for a night followed by a day of activities in nearby Bristol – well, that's what we discovered from the school newsletter. 'Everyone had a wonderful time,' we learnt. Apart from me and Will. Uninvited, there was not even an attempt to include us in the day's activities. Silent in our wheelchairs, we were simply pushed into a different classroom, unaware of the fun we were missing out on.

Fun was not something my primary school were prepared for me to miss. Orienteering, archery, shooting, fencing, canoeing, climbing, biking; every activity my friends did, I joined them for. Not as an onlooker, but as a participant! Having just as much fun as my friends, maybe more...

Determination to include me on the part of the school and the centre meant for the first (and possibly only) time I could feel the breeze in my hair as I sat on Mummy's lap whizzing downhill on an adapted electric bike, the achievement of hitting a bullseye and the exhilarating terror of being hoisted to the top of the climbing wall.

Friends have always been important to me, but my relationship with Will is unique. How can I describe our relationship? Bonded by our similar disabilities, we have never needed words; instead we look deeply into each other's eyes and together we disappear into our fantasies. It was only because of Will that I requested to stay at special school for one afternoon a week, only his company I craved. Despite knowing this, the special school always seemed to find different and separate activities for us to do; if I went to the sensory room, Will was in the classroom, and if Will was chosen to do cooking, I was left in the classroom. Even in the same room, I felt we were deliberately placed apart. Why? No idea, but it made me feel very sad. No amount of protestation from me, Mummy or my carers could change the situation. And it was depressing, watching Will and the other voiceless young people sit in front of animated nursery rhymes, have *The Very Hungry Caterpillar* read to them again and watch lights on the ceiling.

In the end I requested a meeting with the headteacher to explain that I wasn't coming back to special school at the start of the next term. I sat with Mummy and a carer in her airy office with a low coffee table and spelling board between us. I suspect that for the head, this was the first time she had received spelt-out pupil feedback from a child in the PMLD class. Using my spelling board I said, 'Please talk to children like me as you would to an able-bodied child our age.' Her face appeared to contort into barely disguised disbelief. 'And please teach Will to read and write,' I added.

'W e l l,   J o n a t h a n.' The headteacher spoke the most enunciated 'Special' I have ever heard. 'W i l l   h a s   a n   e y e - g a z e   m a c h i n e.   H e   i s   l e a r n i n g   i n   h i s   o w n   w a y.'

Abandoning Will was heartbreaking, but thankfully we could still meet up at the local coffee shop, or at the park where we could sit together, revelling in each other's companionship.

During the next term, I turned ten. Celebrating birthdays is such fun, especially when they are your own; and this one was extra-special because not only was I becoming double figures, I was also able to spell out what I wanted for the first time. From my parents this brought a bread maker, but school's gift to me was unexpected on both sides. In English I was introduced to poetry for the first time. At last, here was a genre that didn't disadvantage my slow speed, where I could play with the sound and meaning of words, to create pictures and emotions, where the perfect fit was the only fit.

On my tenth birthday, having studied William Blake's 'The Tyger' earlier in the week, I spent the morning writing my own birthday poem during my home schooling. Standing at the front of the class in the afternoon, one of my friends read:

Me, Jon-Jon

Jon-Jon! Jon-Jon! Turning ten
In the presence of young men,
What enormous love and joy
Could gift the mighty faithful boy?

Why the sorrow? Why the pain?
Will we celebrate again?
And when earthly time has passed,
What beauty lies? What peace at last?

Jon-Jon! Jon-Jon! Turning ten
In the presence of young men,
What enormous love and joy
Should gift the mighty faithful boy?

It wasn't often that my primary class was
completely silent for a couple of seconds, before
erupting into applause. One TA had to leave the
room, hanky in hand. Reactions like this made
me realise the power of poetry, the mesmerising

effect of the written word and the respect that poetry commands from the listener.

Enriched by the introduction of poetry, life continued with a rhythm of home school, primary school and home. Punctuating this pattern came the eagerly awaited, much-anticipated holidays. Like opening the window on a stuffy day, holidays breathe happiness into our souls.

Excitement for the summer half-term holiday to the coast was mounting to fever pitch, because not only would we visit the beach, we would also be hiring a cottage near our great family friends. With what felt like half the house crammed into my usually spacious van, we set off. But all was not as it should be. For as we drove the considerable distance in the van, I could feel my chest tightening, and this wasn't nervous excitement...

Two days into the week-long holiday, I was wedded to my ventilator, which was turned up to the highest setting possible. While I had no temperature, it seemed that rather than having an infection, my body was giving up. Breathing was increasingly hard work, and as my oxygen supply was increased to silence the saturation monitor, I realised to my delight that this could finally be it. And what perfect timing! With good friends around them, and the beach to escape to, my family was surrounded by love and happiness; I could slip away. So every evening I corralled all my energy to use the spelling board to tell the grown-ups my final words before I went. For Mummy's best friend, I could ask her to look after Mummy when I had gone; for Susannah's best friend I could ask her to stick with my sister through the storms of girls' friendships; for the rest of the family I could share my excitement about going to the garden I had once experienced so clearly, my spiritual home.

One day led intractably to the next. Each morning I would wake to another day in the heart of my family, rather than in the garden. So, the holiday encapsulated my dilemma; to stay or to go. I was so ready to go, but my family will never be as ready as I am.

Returning home on machines and monitors that were usually stowed under the seats, I was beginning to feel a sense of disappointment, in antithesis to my parents' palpable relief. Disappointment that this wasn't the time.

Why hadn't I been called back to the garden?

Why was this not my time?

As well as disappointment, I even felt quite annoyed. From my perspective, everything had been perfect for my departure on holiday. For much as I love my family, my soul yearns to be in the garden forever. So I embody a paradox — happy to be here: sad not to be there. Now I was left with the irksome and slow business of getting better at home, with the knowledge that I would have to go through being that ill again, while the life I couldn't fully join in with continued around me.

Questions turned into prayers, and prayers turned into answers. Time is given as a gift, and gifts should be received with gratitude.

I had been given the extra time so that I could use my voice to make a difference for the voiceless.

CHAPTER EIGHT

PMLD

We are not capable of learning
So do not tell me
There's something going on behind the
   disability.
Treated as useless handicaps
Minds with nothing in there, tragically
Stuck in a wheelchair,
Disabilities visibly crippling –
Just incontinent and dribbling,
We are not

Academically able.

You should make our minds

Stagnate in special education!

We cannot

Learn to read,

Learn to spell,

Learn to write,

Instead let us

Be constrained by a sensory curriculum.

It is not acceptable to say

We have the capacity to learn.

School should occupy us, entertain us; but
   never teach us

You are deluded to believe that

Our education can be looked at another way!

NOW READ IT AGAIN BACKWARDS

A COUPLE OF DAYS LATER, I WAS SAT ON MUMMY'S
LAP WITH SARAH ON THE OTHER SIDE OF THE SPELLING
BOARD. Next to me, washed up and ready to use
again, was my BiPAP ventilator. When recovering
from illness my body even finds breathing
exhausting, so for every hour out of my ventilator
mask, I pay by spending a couple of hours in it.
The longer I spend off it, the more tired I get.
But the mask distorts my view out and, crucially,
for my communication partner, makes it harder
to see where my eyes are looking. Writing is
reduced to a snail's pace, but this conversation is
so important, I must continue.

'There are two ways to do this, Jonathan,' said
Mummy, clearly relieved that I wasn't incessantly
talking about going to the garden anymore. 'You
can write to the minister for education, and you
can approach the media with your story.'

'Let's do both,' I spelt out on my board.

'This is not a good time to go to the media,' she
said. 'In a couple of weeks the nation will vote on
whether we leave the EU, and there will be less
interest or space for stories like yours.'

'Oh.' Those brief exclamations can be so expressive.

'But, on the other hand, you are still very ill, and we don't know how much time you have left.'

So it was that I wrote to the minister and the editors of local and national newspapers, during my home school and afternoon school. On the ventilator, off the ventilator and between sleeps. Nothing could slow me down on my new mission. With a renewed sense of purpose, I sacrificed my limited energy to the cause, using my voice to call for children like me to be taught to read and write.

By mid-June 2016 I had written letters to officials, and the local media had featured my story on their front pages and on the radio. Exposure in the Wiltshire *Gazette & Herald* and the *Wilts & Glos Standard* had Daddy's parishioners handing him the articles neatly cut out and pressed, and a stranger coming up to congratulate me at a village scarecrow event, recognising me from the picture in the paper and saying well done.

After that it went quiet, the pause of a roller coaster carriage before it plunges down the big dipper. Briefly we glimpsed parts of the scenery before we plummeted irreversibly on the adrenalin-fuelled course set before us.

'The cameraman will be here in half an hour,' Mummy said. Since her phone call with the news agency the day before, the pace had been picking up, and now my story was going on the website of the *Mirror* newspaper at lunchtime.

'We need something for people to sign to show their support,' Sarah urged, as the enormity of what was beginning started to sink in.

After a quick phone call for some advice we were racing the clock. This is not how I imagine great campaigns are conceived. With the main body of text lifted from my letter to the minister for education (calling for all disabled children to be taught to read and write regardless of their label), we set to work on a catchy title. Time was ticking on. Succinct and memorable do not come easily to me. Words and phrases were banded around the table, each one tested and checked against the internet. Some good suggestions had already been used.

As the doorbell rang, the campaign 'Teach Us Too' had been born and as midwives, we were ready to introduce it to the cameras. After that short video there were a number of national newspapers which picked up the story; my proudest moment was seeing my poem, 'Song of Voice', printed in *The Times*. Newspapers were being bought on an almost daily basis, and as each one came into the house we all searched for the article and read it. However, when it came to the *Sun*, Mummy inexplicably found the article away from us children and would only present us with the folded page.

'But Mummy, why can't we see the full page he's on?' Susannah couldn't understand it.

'It's a bit rude, darling,' Mummy replied, keeping the paper firmly folded.

'Please, Mummy, it can't be that rude if it's in the paper.'

Earlier that day, when the girls were at school, I had glimpsed the photo next to the article, and now saw my chance to get a better look. While I used my spelling board with a carer to back

Susannah up, Mummy started to give a small boring speech about the different newspapers on sale.

'Are you ready?' Mummy prepared the paper for the big reveal.

Naïve, innocent Susannah could never be ready for this picture... Her arms expanded to make room for her enormous gasp, as her jaw hit the floor.

Tension bristled in the air when the *Mail on Sunday* came to spend the day with us — watching and commentating on my every movement, following me as I went to support Jemima on her sports day, and asking me questions at home. Unlike filming, where the camera is occasionally switched off and everyone can chat off-record, the journalist's notebook was never closed. But it was their coverage that exposed my message to the widest audience.

Now my friends were calling me famous. When *The One Show* covered my story and came to film at school, they became famous too! People started writing me emails from all over the world. Some wrote to say that I was an inspiration, some wrote poems and shared recipes; one lady from Australia even offered to send us some more Lego. Much to our annoyance Mummy wrote back and said we had enough Lego, thank you. Enough Lego? My sisters and I don't believe that is possible, and we were in a grump for the rest of the day. But it was the stories of children like me that kept me focused on making a difference: disabled people whose experience of special school was similar to mine, and parents of disabled children frustrated by a system that wasn't teaching their child to read and write.

Interest in my story was generating enquires not just from journalists from the printed press, but now also from documentary makers. Enjoying the limelight, my instinct was to say 'yes' to everything, but my parents were wisely more cautious and insisted on meeting all the prospective directors and making a final decision as a family. So mealtimes now included discussions on what any documentaries would involve, and the parameters we were happy with. Protecting my sisters from a fly-on-the-wall documentary became the defining factor, for this was their life as well as mine.

When we first met our cameraman/producer, we knew this was a man we would get on well with, who would portray our story with gentleness and humour. Nevertheless, there were real issues with filming me using the spelling board. When my communication partner watches my eyes, they do so from the middle of the board, but the camera angle from the side distorts the correlation between where I am looking and where the communication partner's finger is pointing. To attempt to overcome this issue we tried everything – Sarah with a camera strapped to her forehead, but her forehead not square on; the camera square on but no one pointing where I looked at. Sometimes slowing the film down at least accentuated my eye movements, but then distorted any sounds over the top. In the end a variety of people were filmed using my board in a diverse range of situations – on my comfy seat, otherwise known as Mummy's lap, in my wheelchair at home and at school, with my five carers, my friends at school, Sarah and my mother. In addition, for the final cut, there was not always a direct link between the voiceover and what I was spelling.

Other issues were easier to find solutions for. Who would do the voiceover for the film? While the documentary makers agonised over this, I had the solution and had already asked Lewis, my friend from when I had first started primary school aged four, to be my voice. His abilities in the recording booth surpassed my expectations; his patience with being able to say my words over and over again, and his perseverance in tackling some of the tongue-twisters I had inadvertently put into the script, were second to none. At the end of a long day's recording, when we were all tired having just listened to him working so hard, Lewis was still able to crack a joke.

So it was that the cameraman followed me during November and December 2016. During that time, I also found myself at the Department for Education in London seated opposite the then Minister of State for Vulnerable Children and Families, Edward Timpson, who had responsibility for special education.

Change is easy to talk about but almost impossible to achieve. Like a pincer movement, I have tried to focus my energies on those at the top (policymakers) and those at the delivery end (teachers and trainers) in the hope that I can make a difference for the children caught in the middle. Setting off before dawn to meet Mr Timpson, Daddy gave a running commentary into a video camera for most of the journey amid Mummy's protestations. And, as the sun rose, reflected on London's iconic landmarks, anticipation for what lay ahead hung in my silent contemplation.

'I have come as a voice for the voiceless.' I spelled out my rehearsed line for the minister, feeling the weight of all those I represented on my shoulders.

Next to me on the table sat a box containing the signatures of over 180,000 supporters of my petition, outlining my dream that every non-verbal child should be taught to read and write in school, regardless of their label. Nervous excitement for this moment had robbed me of most of the night's sleep, and now I felt so small and insignificant. How could a child in a wheelchair hope to make a difference? And yet, this is what I believe that I was given extra time to do. Often when people talk with me they can't help but look at the person sounding out the letters and words I spell. Not so with Mr Timpson. As I spoke with him, he looked at me intently and I felt my words were falling on receptive ears.

'Today's a chance for us to learn more about what we can do,' he said. 'I think it's really important that no one has barriers put in their way.'

Not only were we talking about the challenges of effecting change on the ground, but we had both brought experts to the meeting. I was accompanied by experts in the field of literacy teaching for students like me using augmentative and alternative communication (AAC), and Mr Timpson's top special educational needs advisor joined the discussion. Once the cameras left the room, the real business of discussing change took place.

'What you've shown me through coming here today is that you have some very strong and passionate views that you want to share,' said Mr Timpson, 'and the more that we can educate teachers as well as everybody else, the advantages that has, not just for them but also for their pupils. Then we will have done a good thing and you will have made something important happen.'

Thus, we left with promises of some research to be commissioned into the literacy teaching of children like me, and the feeling that my message had been understood. But in its delivery I had spent myself, so in antithesis to the elation of the rest of my group of supporters and experts, I felt an exhausted flatness.

Gaining momentum, my campaign was beginning to attract the attention of a wide audience. Not long after my article in the *Guardian* was published in January 2017, Mummy got a phone call that Susannah overheard. After sharing the news with Daddy and me, we were instructed not to tell anyone else...

Six weeks later in May, my seven-year-old Susannah had turned eight, and had still not told a soul. Travelling to London with anticipation buzzing in the van, Mummy and Daddy sent the emails I had prepared the day before, and the congratulations started to fizz into our excited bubble. St James' Palace. An invitation from St James' Palace to receive an award from none other than Princes William and Harry to commemorate their mother, Princess Diana. An inaugural Diana Legacy Award. How I wish we had cleaned the van before its dirty country high-tide marks featured in the foreground of any tourist photos of the palace that day. Wheeled from grime to grandeur!

It was one of those days when, looking back, it seems like a surreal dream; but unlike a dream, I can relive the moment I chatted with Prince Harry and received the award from the princes by looking back at the footage and photos. But those photos belie my happiness. When I am tense with excitement or nerves or both, my cerebral palsy tenses my body too. Strong spasms pull my muscles tight and smiling becomes impossible. Inside I am happy and excited, from the outside I look at best indifferent and at worst miserable. Like a sponge my body soaks up the atmosphere of the room, so it was only at the end of the ceremony when the room erupted into prolonged applause that my body relaxed and realigned itself to give my muscles the tone to slip off Mummy's knee. With her supporting me I stood on my feet and whooped with joy. Out of the corner of my eye, I saw Prince Harry smile across at my mother – obviously relieved that I had enjoyed it after all. Saying it was an honour doesn't do it justice, especially when I met the other young people from around the world getting the same award as me, all working towards making the world a better place.

Big days come with a health price for me, and at home that evening I paid it. As a reminder from my body that my chance to make a difference is limited, I had a seizure.

With Teach Us Too morphing from one child's campaign to a movement making links with other people and organisations, it was becoming clear that it was coming of age. I am more than Teach Us Too and Teach Us Too is more than me. So now, when I am asked to speak in public, I do so as Jonathan Bryan, blogger at Eye Can Talk, championing the message of Teach Us Too. It also means that when I breathe my last, Teach Us Too will live on.

Now, rather than spending my free time writing emails and making connections, I can concentrate on my writing: poetry, and even a speech for the House of Lords, which I gave at a Diana Award reception there in September 2017:

I received the Legacy Award in recognition of my Teach Us Too campaign for all children to be taught to read and write, regardless of their label.

It was an immense honour to receive this award remembering Princess Diana, who so often went out of her way to show solidarity with those society would rather forget about.

Her legacy award has given me a stronger platform on which I am a voice for the voiceless. My dream is a special education system where academic competence is assumed, rather than assumptions about academic ability based on physical disability. Unfortunately, current education policy is tipping the other way, with proposals from the Rochford Review that schools will no longer need to report to government on children labelled with profound and multiple learning difficulties (as I was). This is against a backdrop where special schools are increasingly opting for non-subject-specific learning; i.e., literacy teaching is no longer required. This lack of accountability signals that the education of children like me is of very little importance. Imagine Ofsted was abolished in mainstream education, because no one really cared what children were taught in schools. Yet this is what is happening to children like me in education.

If my mother hadn't removed me from special school for a few hours a day to teach me to read and write I would not be able to write this for you today. For a non-verbal child, learning to read and write is not just a life skill. It unlocks our voice. It gives us life in all its fullness. I am not unique. There are more children like me in special school who need an education system that believes they are worth teaching too. Then my story of learning to write and communicate will not be so unique either.

I don't have much time left, so I am asking you to get behind my campaign and use your influence to ensure there is accountability and aspiration for children who are often marginalised and judged.

My body is very weak, but my desire to make a difference for children like me is very strong.

With Diana's legacy I am building my own.

Sometimes my spelling board is too slow for the moment. Written over three mornings, my speech was read out by my nervous mother to a packed room of lords, ladies and MPs. My turn to be proud of her! Afterwards many people congratulated us both, and new connections were made for my campaign.

When I write and spell, people listen. Like the moment the expectant crowd hush to watch the tennis player serve, the atmosphere when I 'speak' concentrates into the moment, and I hold the attention of my audience.

I often need to rely on those around me to read out my words. One other such occasion was the premiere of my CBBC programme, *My Life: Locked-in Boy*. Transforming the school into a prestigious venue for the screening, my friends, family and esteemed guests wore their party best to walk the red carpet and join me for the event. Valiant Susannah read my speech for the evening. Standing in front of an audience of over 100 people, my slight Susannah opened her mouth and astounded everyone. Not only could we all hear every word projected to the back, but she delivered the speech with such presence, aplomb and panache, while I watched her with pride in my heart and a smile on my face.

With the completion of one project, I could refocus on another... the writing of this book.

Spelling and writing is slow and intentional; giving voice to my thoughts is a measured activity. For writing, this means sitting in the moment I am describing — seeing it, hearing it, feeling it. Words swirl onto the page, portraying the experience to be relived by my reader. Words that need shepherding, culling, matching before being committed to a piece.

As a budding writer, I now appreciated the great oaks of English literature even more — Shakespeare's sonnets, Wordsworth's poetry, Tolkien's *The Hobbit*. Not just as the reader, but as a writer I could admire the techniques and language in new ways. And there is one modern author I aspire to be like the most... Michael Morpurgo. He paints his imagery using words as his brush; scenes are described in vivid detail while not holding up the unfurling plot, so the reader is immersed and travels the story with the characters.

Hearing *Kensuke's Kingdom* in our van as we drove
to and from Norfolk, our first family introduction
to Morpurgo was impressive. What other author
can hold the attention of a pre-schooler and a
grandmother? For the first time on holiday no
one minded long journeys if we could listen to
his words, and trips in the van were almost sought
after. Following that trip, to my delight, we studied
Why the Whales Came at primary school, and my love
of Morpurgo's writing was established. The more
I read, the more I tried to emulate his writing, and
the more I longed to meet the man behind the
books. So Sarah applied to the UK charity Make-
A-Wish for my dream to become a reality. Dreams
coming true is what Make-A-Wish specialise in,
and thus in December 2016 I was sat in a room at
Exeter Cathedral waiting to meet my literary hero
before he performed his story, *The Best Christmas
Present in the World.* Christmas magic filled the air at
the event, held to raise money for Mr Morpurgo's
charity, Farms for City Children.

Anticipation electrified the room, magnifying
every small noise as we waited for the great man

himself. After a number of false starts and the ticking by of too many minutes, the door handle depressed and in he came; sporting his signature red coat, a jaunty black beret and a warm, genuine smile.

'Hallo Jonathan, you came all this way. All this way just to shake an old man's hand. Do you know how lucky you are to be ten? Ten's young! Seventy-three's old!'

Drawing his chair close to mine, we had an initial discussion about his writing before I handed him my story, *Curtains to Freedom*.

'Can I read this aloud?' Mr Morpurgo asked. My story read aloud by the master himself? I can't believe he needed to ask!

'"Listening, looking, and wanting to be heard, I spend my time unable to tell my story. In silence, I live behind the curtains…"'

As Michael took my hand, we lost ourselves in the richness of his narration. Transporting us past the confines of the room where we had met, we travelled behind the curtains of my silence together.

When he had finished the story, he clapped. 'It's remarkable writing. You use words like a paintbrush, and also like a composer. This is extraordinary. I think this needs to be sent to the minister for education. People should see this! My goodness me, what thoughts go on in that head?'

As the master of modern atmospheric story-telling, Mr Morpurgo is my literary hero. To hear him utter these words after reading my story was the biggest compliment I could ever hope for.

'I am your student,' I spelt out.

'That's lovely,' he said. 'I've always wanted a student! This is very strong in emotion, this is deeply felt, and I think maybe that is what links your writing to mine. I *try* to make my stories full of the feeling that I have inside me; sometimes it's anger, sometimes it's love, it can be all sorts of things. So we're linked that way I think – you, me...' ever the dramatist, he completed the triptych with '...and Shakespeare.' Laughter rippled through the room with his final flourish. 'I don't really like meeting writers who are every bit as good as me... particularly when they're younger than me!'

'I've very much enjoyed meeting a writer older than me,' I spelt back with a grin.

Sitting back in his chair, Mr Morpurgo looked at me and said, 'I'm not often speechless Jonathan, but I sort of am.'

Listening to Michael's Christmas story at Exeter Cathedral was beautiful; his turn to transport me to another time and place. Afterwards he asked if I had enjoyed the performance.

'You are compelling,' I spelt.

'You always come out with surprising words,' he said, and laughed. 'Lovely, Jonathan. I've so loved meeting you. You've made my evening.'

To my delight I continued to 'meet' Mr Morpurgo in his many books, which I read at home and studied at school. Through all the activity, excitement and busy-ness of campaigning, it was school that kept me grounded. Not treated differently, I loved being as normal a student as I could; when we did experiments I joined in, when we played cricket I held the bat with my carer and was propelled full speed in my wheelchair, and when I misbehaved I got told off! Like my peers at primary school, I took my SATs exams at the end of Year 6, with some extra time to compensate for my slow eye pointing. Usually I love a test, but I found the stress of public exams very hard work, and the accumulation of tests day after day exhausting. Sometimes being a 'normal' student is less enjoyable, but as Mummy often reminds me: I can't have my cake and eat it!

Leaving primary school was sad. As a school, they had travelled my communication and education journey with me: believing in me, nurturing me and teaching me. Friends I had known since I was four, and played with every day, were not all going on to my next school. But the end of one era of my life heralded the beginning of the next. In September I began at our local mainstream secondary school, studying English, maths, science and DT.

For me, the climax of being able to spell has

not been education or campaigning, or awards. The pinnacle of my journey with speech has been the ability to share my faith. When I started to spell, words didn't alter my faith, but sharing it using words changed the perceptions of those around me. So when I got the opportunity to be confirmed by the Bishop of Swindon in Malmesbury Abbey, I jumped at the chance. For now, I didn't just walk with Jesus, I publicly joined the throng on the shared adventure.

During the service my godfather read my words — my testimony to everything that has gone before and all that lies ahead — which I had called 'Living Life in all its Fullness':

> With Jesus as my saviour, companion and friend, I have lived my hours here with happiness in my spirit and contented calm in my soul. Knowing Jesus is with me, cradling me in pain, sheltering me from darkness and beckoning me forward, has given me the strength and serenity to look life in the eye and smile. Like the

constancy of the second hand of a clock, Jesus inhabits the quaver beats of my life; and as that beat slows, I look forward with excited anticipation to the day I will see Jesus and live together with him in the garden forever. In the meantime, I cleave to Jesus: my faith and my life.

Like my life expectancy, this book is short. But why did I write it in the first place? To answer that, I need to transport you back. Before my wish was granted, before Michael Morpurgo had met me in person, I, like thousands of others, wrote him a fan letter. Having read his book *Cool!* about a boy in a coma, I explained that the story was very different from my own particular experience of being unable to speak. I sent him my poem 'Song of Silence', and wrote: 'I have a story I must share with you, a sad story, where children like me are trapped inside because no one has unlocked their voice.' Asking him to write a story about non-verbal disabled children like me, I sent my letter – hoping for, but never expecting, a reply.

Many months later I received a wonderful handwritten postcard from Michael Morpurgo, suggesting I read *Listen to the Moon* and telling me: 'As for writing a story with non-verbal disabled children, this is for you to do, when you feel the moment is right. It is your story. Tell it.'

EPILOGUE

AS A VOICE FOR THE VOICELESS, I HAVE WRITTEN THIS BOOK FOR THOSE WHO CAN'T YET READ AND WRITE. As I said in my speech at the House of Lords reception, for non-verbal children, learning to read and write is not just a life skill. It unlocks our voice. It gives us life in all its fullness. Stagnating in an educational stalemate, their story is waiting to be told. My proceeds from the sale of this book will go towards my Teach Us Too charity (www.teachustoo.org.uk), which is working towards the literacy teaching of all children regardless of their label.

Last week my best friend Will came to visit me, and Mummy asked him if he would like to try using my spelling board. Using his high-tech eye-gaze machine, Will had become proficient at communicating by choosing pictures with words underneath, from a selection offered to him. To my knowledge, though, he hadn't used a spelling board or been taught how to read. Everything he wrote that day was from self-taught, whole-word reading from the options presented on his eye-gaze machine. Just like me, Will is labelled with having profound and multiple learning difficulties, but despite his label, and never having been taught to read, he was able to use my spelling board. With my board in front of him, Will looked at the top right-hand square, followed by the red square.

Mummy sounded out the vowel he had chosen. Having spent the last two and a half years watching me use my spelling board, Will was decisive in his choice, but now he paused, uncertain.

Then Mummy offered: '"i". Or it could be an "I".'

At which point Will continued with, 'don't want to go home.'

Thus I witnessed Will's first free conversation with the board; his first words, his first 'I love you' to his mother, aged 13. Will can't be the last. But the last words of my story will be his:

'Give the spelling to more people.'

Going Home

Go my soul and go my eyes,
Onwards, onwards through fateful times,
Lift me, lift me home.
I must travel on.
Travel on.

Beckoning, calling, summoning, coaxing,
Drawing me homewards.
Homewards.
Travelling time on the wings of hope.
Fly my soul. Fly.

Anticipate home, yearn only for home,
Traversing on, voyaging on, journeying on.
Soar my soul, soar,
Steady my eyes. Steer steady.

Alone with Him in my heart,
Over the youngest years, through the
sleeplessness,
She my soul-mate joins me.
Together, our souls glide on.
Glide on.

Eyes sickening, body weakening, lungs dying,
Be strong my soul.
Be strong.
Falling, failing, fading...

Eyes glimpsing home.
Safe, warm, free, secure,
Soul's rest.
Eyes discerning, eyes burning,
Dragged back, hauled back.
Next time.

Silence.
Soul's suffocating silence.
Eyes searching onwards, upwards,
Trapped.
Until, until...

...I look out and see,
Eyes discerning, fingers pointing, letters
spelling,
Break free my soul,
Break free.

Onwards, eyes dancing soul's beat,
Dance on my eyes.
Beat on my soul.
Home is calling, beckoning,
Soul's yearning home.

ABOUT TEACH US TOO

A portion of the proceeds from the sale of this book will be donated to Jonathan Bryan's Teach Us Too charity.

Teach Us Too hopes to further the aims of Jonathan's ongoing petition, which he presented to the Minister of State for Vulnerable Children and Families at the Department of Education in 2016 — to promote the teaching of literacy to *all* children regardless of their label. Following that meeting, the department commissioned and published some research into literacy support for children and young people who use augmentative and alternative communication (AAC). The task is a big one and requires a shift in perceptions of what is possible, but with Jonathan as Teach Us Too's patron, the charity is determined to make a difference. Jonathan has driven this campaign, and his charity will surely be his lasting legacy.

Please visit www.teachustoo.org.uk to find out more about the charity, its aims and how you can support it.